Diets Make You Fat
Eating Makes You Skinny

by
Dr. Rafael Bolio

Bloomington, IN  Milton Keynes, UK

AuthorHouse™
1663 Liberty Drive, Suite 200
Bloomington, IN 47403
www.authorhouse.com
Phone: 1-800-839-8640

AuthorHouse™ UK Ltd.
500 Avebury Boulevard
Central Milton Keynes, MK9 2BE
www.authorhouse.co.uk
Phone: 08001974150

© 2006 Dr. Rafael Bolio. All rights reserved.

No part of this book may be reproduced, stored in a retrieval system, or transmitted by any means without the written permission of the author.

First published by AuthorHouse 10/30/2006

ISBN: 1-4259-7381-7 (sc)

Library of Congress Control Number: 2006909408

Printed in the United States of America
Bloomington, Indiana

This book is printed on acid-free paper.

Table of Contents

PROLOGUE	vii
INTRODUCTION	xi
PART ONE — UNDERSTANDING BODY FAT	**1**
1. Why Do Diets Make You Fat?	3
2. Finding the Real Causes of Excess Body Fat	8
3. Excess Body Fat as a Result of Overeating	10
4. Excess Body Fat Due to Eating Between Meals	12
5. Excess Body Fat Due to Heredity	13
6. Excess Body Fat Due to Emotional Factors	16
7. Excess Body Fat Due to Excess Fat in the Diet	19
8. Excess Body Fat and Carbohydrates	25
9. Summary: the Causes of Excess Body Fat	31
PART TWO — REDUCING EXCESS BODY FAT	**33**
10. The Diet-Disaster Phenomenon	35
11. Walking: the Perfect Exercise	38
12. The Myth of the Scale	42
13. The Way You Eat Is More Important than What You Eat	48
14. Choose Wisely	51
15. How To Reduce or Avoid Excess Body Fat	58
16. Eating Without Discomfort	60
17. Preparing To Change the Way You Eat	65
PART THREE — THE BOLIO SYSTEM	**69**
Week One	71
Week Two	83
Week Three	91
Week Four	111
Week Five	118
Week Six	125
Week Seven	132

Week Eight	139
Week Nine?	150
The Last Week	156

PART FOUR   ANY QUESTIONS? 159
The Plateau	161
Questions and Answers	164

APPENDIX   SERVINGS LIST   183

Prologue

Whatever happened to the simple things of life?

It used to be that being chubby was healthy and that parents would do almost anything to make their babies gain weight.

Then suddenly excess body fat became one of America's worst health problems.

Now being hungry is "in," and eating is "out."

In America, where there's enough food for everyone, almost four out of ten adults are dieting, eating less than they should and/or less than they want to.

Many years ago, when parents were trying to make their children gain weight, being overweight was quite unusual. Now that everyone is trying to lose weight, the number of people with excess weight is on the rise. If current trends continue, by the year 2050 more than 90% of Americans will be overweight and/or obese.

Excess body fat has now become everyone's problem.

And when we study *why* people gain weight, things get very, very complicated.

MYTHS

As you read this book, you will discover that most of what has been said about why you gain weight is more myth than fact.

First of all, there is no relationship between how much you eat and how much you weigh. Some eat great quantities, others eat normally, many are permanently on diet and yet excess body fat persists in all of them.

Also, it turns out that the metabolisms of overweight and thin are identical, as long as neither of them goes on a diet.

What about exercise? By exercising, you can lose up to ten pounds and reduce health damage caused by to excess weight. But if you have more than ten pounds to lose, you'd better start looking for other options. Furthermore, the overweight are not lazy as everyone assumes, since when they walk, they use the same energy as thin people who *run*. Those who are overweight are constantly exercising even when sitting or sleeping, since their excess weight increases their workload for ***any type of activity***.

We cannot leave behind myths surrounding food groups; i.e. we're fat because of sugars, fats, and/or protein. Here you will discover that virtually everything you have heard or believed about food groups is false.

Worse still, although almost everyone in America is on diet, or has been on diet, long-term results are extremely disappointing, since 95% will regain any weight lost through dieting and/or exercise.

Furthermore, despite the fact that scientists have known of these dismal results for years, more than 90 billion dollars are still spent yearly in the United States on obesity treatments. If you have 90 billion dollars in your pocket, use them on something else, since long term weight-loss treatments only give you less than 5% of probability for succeeding.

A SIMPLER SOLUTION

To obtain permanent weight loss, many changes must be made in the way you treat it.

Here you will learn how to change the way you eat, and not what you eat or how much you eat, to win this battle.

No magical remedies are promised. Excess body fat is lost very, very slowly. Nor can I promise that the program presented in this book (the Bolio System) is a walk in the park. Without discipline, there is no possibility of success. And even with discipline, 15 percent will not obtain the results they want. Does it surprise you that I will admit that my program will not work for everyone? Should you buy some other book that can offer better results instead? No. There are no better books. Traditional low-calorie diets fail to make you lose weight in more than 20% of the time, and the other diet books don't tell you that, do they?

The greatest difference between the Bolio System and other programs is that you will lose excess fat through eating more, not eating less. If you are already eating well, you do not have to reduce your food intake; just learn to eat in a different way.

In order for this program to work, the way you have always thought about food must be challenged. Specifically, you must understand that accumulation of body fat is more a result of how we think than of how we eat. This will become very clear once you start this plan, since you will be eating all food groups in abundance and losing excess fat.

Information and recommendations in this book are intended for a general audience. Even though this book will help anyone lose excess body fat, it provides general information that does not replace consultation with your doctor. If you are obese, remember that it is a disease, and as such must be attended by a doctor. It does not mean that you cannot follow current recommendations; you just have to do this under medical supervision.

I strongly insist that, before applying this or any other program that changes eating patterns, you get a physical checkup and the approval of your doctor, even if you are not overweight or obese.

I am a registered doctor in Mexico, where I have been successfully treating people with excess body weight since 1980. However in the United States of America I am not claiming to offer medical services of any kind but simply sharing my experience through this book.

In 1990, I began working with the Mexican government in a national program which recommended a balanced diet as one of the primary tools to improve health. Nutritional recommendations in this program were in agreement with recommendations of major medical societies such as the American Heart Association, the American Cancer Society and the American Diabetes Association. This project showed me that anyone can improve his or her health through eating, as long as it is done with a sensible strategy.

The Bolio System presented in this book is based on what I learned from that project. It includes very simple menus that will help you shed excess fat. All of these menus are based on the guidelines of medical societies cited above.

In order for this program to work for you, you must first change the way you think and the way you feel about food. If you allow this to happen, excess body fat can certainly be eradicated from your life.

Introduction

Excess body fat is a problem that has been treated and mistreated by many, many self-appointed "experts". Mothers, cousins, brothers, shamans, psychics, and even a well-intentioned friend or two have tried to cure it without success. Everyone knows about a magical technique that makes you quickly lose weight, but no one seems to know how to keep those pounds off permanently.

The number of weight-loss programs is indeed impressive.

The best known is EOH (Eat Only Half), which means that you should eat half as much as you are used to eating.

Or, if you prefer, you can choose the very popular diet that eliminates all or most carbohydrates (sugars) from the menu. According to the experts who advocate this diet, sugar consumption is the true cause of excess weight; they recommend that you reduce or eliminate sugars and eat all the protein and fat that you want in order to lose your excess body fat.

In opposition to these experts, there are other experts who swear by carbohydrates and argue that excess body weight is really caused by the fat that you eat. Therefore, they advise that for the rest of your life you should eat all the food groups that followers of the low-carb diets avoid; fruit, bread, pasta, beans, potatoes and avoid fat in the diet, which means that you must eat skinless boiled chicken breast, tuna canned in water, lettuce, and tomatoes.

Then there are programs that make it even more complicated and recommend that you eat certain foods during precisely-defined hours of the day, arguing that fruits ingested in the afternoon or combined with meat definitely make you fat.

Those trying to shed pounds and inches are certainly confronted by an immense array of possibilities. What is most frustrating and confusing is that these programs often contradict each other. More confusing still, when you follow the recommendations of **any** of these diets, no matter how bizarre, you will certainly lose weight.

But let me also make this perfectly clear: No matter what program you follow, the excess weight you lose will almost always return. Those who market weight-loss programs may whisper sweet words in your ear, but the truth is that diets do not eradicate excess body fat. They definitely make you lose inches and weight, but there is no way that they will keep fat from coming back.

Then what sense is there in my writing another weight loss book?

The situation is not hopeless. There is a solution. Excess weight can be eliminated. Fortunately, the solution is found in what is most feared but always longed for; food!

This book will help you to permanently lose excess fat by eating all food groups in abundance. But in order for this to happen, you must first erase from your mind ideas that have damaged instead of helping, and exchange them for new and useful information. This new knowledge will help you eat without fear.

This book is divided into four parts:

The first section analyzes why strict diets don't work, and how they may even lead to greater accumulation of body fat. This section also explains the real reasons body fat increases.

The second section presents proven ways that excess body fat can be eliminated.

The third section presents the Bolio System, which will teach you how to eat as much as you want of any food group and remain slender. These recommendations are ideal for those who can prepare their meals at home. If you frequently eat in restaurants, I recommend my other book, *What the Naturally Skinny Do to Stay Skinny*.

The last section answers frequently asked questions about how to apply the Bolio System.

This is very important: before applying recommendations, carefully read this book at least three times. This way you will understand why one must eat to lose excess fat and why other methods have proven useless and even counterproductive.

More information can be found on my website: www.drbolio.com or www.esbelto.com (Spanish version).

PART ONE
UNDERSTANDING BODY FAT

1. Why Do Diets Make You Fat?

Once you develop excess body fat, it is extremely difficult to eradicate it. Multiple clinical studies show truly disappointing long-term results. The most you can expect to obtain from a diet is a ten-pound reduction one year after starting it, even if during the first months you lost greater amounts. By two years, in all likelihood, not only will you have returned to your initial weight, but you will have gained even more.

You must understand this fundamental principle: **Restricting the amount of food you eat (going on a diet) does not permanently eliminate excess body fat.**

Severely restricted weight-loss diets have been widely criticized, since scientific studies have proven them to be of little use. It is true that eating less makes you lose weight, but this does not protect you from regaining lost weight when you go back to your normal eating pattern.

Even more discouraging are recent reports that reveal how continuously losing and regaining weight (the yo-yo syndrome) curtails longevity. These studies show that in the long run intermittent weight loss can cause more damage than being overweight. Dieting is definitely a very risky matter.

Nowadays, it is well known that very low calorie diets will not eradicate excess body fat and may even increase it. In order to understand why this happens, we need to take into account that we have already faced food scarcity for thousands of years.

The human body is extraordinary and has the ability to adapt to severe environmental changes. We have survived for thousands of years under the coldest and hottest conditions. We are one of the few living organisms that can flourish in almost every corner of the earth. In order to survive in a desert, a jungle, or a polar region, facing dramatic changes in climate and available food, we developed metabolic survival mechanisms.

Specifically, nature has provided us with biological defenses to ensure survival in situations of food scarcity. Those who try to lose weight by eating less do not know or forget these biologic adaptations. There is nothing new under the sun when it comes to restricting food intake, and our body knows what to do when this happens; it stores fat!

I will describe some of these adaptations. Don't be concerned if they seem overly technical. Metabolic changes are very complex, very difficult to understand, and even more difficult to explain. What is important is that you understand in general why diets don't work. Following are some of the changes which occur:

1. The ***digestive tract*** increases in size and weight and in the number of its villi (hair like projections from the walls of the canal which absorb food passing through). That is, the stomach enlarges so that it will accommodate more food and whatever is eaten will be more easily absorbed. Contrary to popular belief, diets make your stomach larger, not smaller.

2. The body increases its production of ***lipoprotein lipase***, an enzyme which makes it easier to store dietary fat by forcing the body's cells to absorb as much fat as possible.

3. The body produces more "***reverse T3***." Normally, the human body produces the hormone T4 and then converts some of the T4 into another hormone, T3; both regulate the body's metabolism. During starvation (dieting), T4 is converted into "reverse T3" (a mirror image of the hormone T3), which is metabolically inactive. This reduces the basal metabolism and the ability of muscle tissues to consume fat. This reaction also occurs in response to infectious disease.

4. The tone of the ***sympathetic nervous system*** decreases, leading to fat being stored around the waist and upper body. The sympathetic nervous system regulates what is often termed the "fight or flight" response. It accelerates the heart rate, widens the bronchial tubes, decreases movement of the large intestine, constricts blood vessels, dilates the pupils, activates goose bumps, triggers sweating, raises blood pressure and increases the metabolism. All these events take up energy, and when they are decreased, the body reduces its energy expenditure.

5. The thermogenic response (***luxusconsumption***) is decreased. That is, the body loses its ability to convert into heat any excess food that is eaten. As a result, overeating more easily leads to an increase in excess body fat.

6. **Brown fat** tissue becomes less active. Brown fat burns fat to produce heat. It is also believed that it establishes how efficiently the body utilizes its own fat stores. Therefore, more fat is kept within the body.

7. The body **starts eating its own muscle tissue** weeks before it utilizes fat stores. The human body has been programmed to protect fat stores over muscle mass, since body fat is more important for survival. The energy that a body spontaneously generates (the basal metabolic rate) is directly related to the amount of muscle tissue. Therefore, less muscle means a lower metabolic rate.

8. The body's **basal metabolism** decreases; that is, all body activities are slowed down–physical, mental, and sexual. The first activity altered, in a matter of minutes, is the intellectual function; multiple studies have demonstrated that skipping breakfast, even for one day, will reduce scholastic achievement at any age, as well as the ability to perform complex manual activities.

If it were not for the above mentioned changes, the human race would never have survived through centuries of difficult circumstances. Nature's greatest gift to humanity is not the brain; it is the fat cell.

We are blessed with these extraordinary adaptations to food scarcity (or even total absence of food) from the first day we are born. In fact, newborn babies have enough fat to survive for days without food: In 1985, when Mexico City was hit by one of its worst earthquakes in modern history, a maternity ward with newborn babies in it was completely demolished. Fortunately, some rain fell during the following days, and this allowed the newborns to drink water by sucking the debris that was around them. By the time rescue teams found them under the debris, many of these babies had survived for weeks on only the water that they were able to drink.

All of these changes are classified as metabolic adaptations for survival. Very low calorie diets will activate precisely these defense mechanisms, putting the body into "*starvation mode*."

Moreover, the changes described above are only biological adaptations to food deprivation. Many more mechanisms are triggered in the behavioral, emotional, and social spheres. These reactions are identical in overweight and thin people who reduce their food intake.

Anyone who has been on a diet for more than a year may not be aware of the metabolic changes that have taken place in his body, but he is definitely conscious of what happens in the long term. That is, he knows that after a certain time (between three and six months), weight loss will slow down, and sooner or later (about a year) he will regain all the weight he has lost, even though he continues to follow his strict diet. Worse still, if he leaves the diet, he will gain more fat than he had lost.

Reducing food intake transforms the body into an extraordinary food-saving machine! Thus, far from preventing obesity, strict weight-loss diets favor its increase.

In other words, diets make you fat.

Therefore, regaining weight has little to do with lack of will power. In fact, the stricter the diet, i.e. the stronger the will power, the higher the possibility of gaining more weight than was lost in the first place. When you go on a strict diet, you're not struggling against poor will power or addiction to food, but against natural changes triggered by eating less. This is a struggle where you have little possibility of winning.

To free yourself from excess fat, you don't need a miracle plan or a magic method, but prudence and knowledge. Going on a diet without knowledge is foolish and can cause more damage than being overweight itself.

Don't be fooled by the immediate effects of diets. Eating less or eliminating some food group from your menu will certainly make you lose weight and inches in the short run. However, as you continue, organic changes in your body will slow down this weight loss, and eventually the body's ability to accumulate fat will be triggered. That is why, at the end of two years of dieting, not only will you return to your initial weight, but you may even weigh more.

People on diet, lose muscle, water, patience, and poise, but fat returns and even increases, causing frustration.

It may surprise you that excess body fat must be treated with a sufficient and balanced diet, but it is true. The good news is that eating will make you skinny. Those who refuse to eat will continue to have excess body fat for the rest of their lives or end up with severe problems as a consequence of surgery, drugs, or their intermittent dieting.

2. Finding the Real Causes of Excess Body Fat

There is no medical problem surrounded by such ignorance, errors, and inappropriate treatment as excess body fat. For many years, the medical community steadfastly clung to outdated theories that, far from helping patients, confused and harmed them.

A very clear example is the myth of food. Years ago, medical students viewed excess body fat as a natural variation of the human body, similar to height or the color of the skin. They were taught that excess body fat was due to excessive eating, that it could be solved by eating less, and that overweight people were not cured because they did not stick to their diets. Medical students were also taught that most people were unable to stick to their diets because they were addicted to food. This made the doctor's position simple: If the problem was solved, it was because of the diet prescribed by the doctor, and if it wasn't solved, it was because of the patient, who did not follow the doctor's orders.

For years, excess body fat was not viewed as a health problem, and therefore medical societies did not challenge the questionable concepts of self-appointed experts that, far from helping overweight people, confused and harmed them. Weight management was even viewed by doctors as a vanity issue, something like going to get your hair cut. Those health professionals who did treat patients with excess body fat were often ridiculed by their peers.

It was not until 1984 that excess body fat was internationally accepted as having adverse effects on health and longevity. This happened after the National Health Institute promoted a Consensus Development Conference on Obesity. The results were published in February 1985. The panel of experts concluded that excess weight was clearly associated with hypertension, high cholesterol levels, heart disease, higher incidence of diabetes, certain cancers, and other medical problems. Thus, excess body fat is one of the youngest diseases in the history of medicine. It has always been with us, but it was not until 1985 that scientists finally demonstrated that it is a real threat to our health.

This consensus led to a number of original and extremely revealing studies that helped explain why excess body fat appears. At present, the scientific community recognizes that most of the old ideas concerning the causes of excess body fat are more myth than truth. The real causes of this problem are now better established, as well as the best ways to solve it.

Unfortunately there are many overweight people who are not aware of recent scientific findings and still believe old and outdated theories. They focus their efforts on maintaining their will power, convince themselves that they really are addicted to food, and pass the rest of their lives applying techniques that will never solve their problem.

It is very important that you understand the true reasons for the accumulation of excess fat within the body. Carefully read the following chapters. Then read them again, as many times as necessary, until you are sure you understand them. Only then will you be prepared to reject magic cures and take the proper steps to lose, and keep off, excess body fat.

3. Excess Body Fat as a Result of Overeating

One of the most popular and false ideas is that the only way you can get fat is by eating more than your body requires. According to this idea, two plus two equals four. In nature, things are seldom that simple.

In fact, current findings are quite surprising. No scientific study has demonstrated a direct relationship between total calorie ingestion and excess body weight. It is false to state that excess body fat is only caused by overeating.

In 1982, the research scientist Aida Thompson analyzed studies of food consumption among overweight and thin. Six studies showed that there were no differences; five showed that the overweight ate less, and only two found that overweight individuals ate more than thin individuals.

In 1989, the research scientist Judith Rodin presented twenty-three more studies that showed no difference between the quantity of food eaten by overweight people and the quantity of food eaten by thin people.

Those studies that did report overweight individuals eating more than slender individuals did not find a relationship between how much they ate and how much they weighed.

Some eat a great deal, others eat moderate quantities, and many eat very little, but the problem of excess body fat persists among all of them.

We do not always gain fat by eating in excess. Overeating has been a natural tendency for thousands of years, and consequently nature has gifted us with defense mechanisms that prevent weight gain when we eat more than our body needs. The body usually transforms excess food into heat, not into fat. This process is called luxusconsumption or thermogenesis. That is why there is no relationship between the quantity of food eaten and the degree of excess body weight.

There is a technique called the doubly labeled water method (DLW), which was developed by Nathan Lifson in the early 1950s. DLW, in essence, turns the body into its own metabolic recorder. After a loading of water labeled with deuterium and ^{18}O, the deuterium washes out of the body as water, and the ^{18}O washes out of the body as water and carbon dioxide. The difference between the two elimination rates is used to measure energy expenditure (how much energy we use up in 24 hours). DLW studies carried out on overweight subjects have shown that they misreport what and how much they eat by up to 50%. But when we compare quantities that overweight individuals and thin individuals eat, it turns out that both usually take the same amount of calories (2000 to 2500).

Obese individuals will almost always eat more that what they believe they are eating, but even so, they are ingesting similar quantities as non obese individuals.

Anyone who insists obesity is only secondary to overeating does not have the slightest idea of why excess body fat exists.

Although obesity does not exist where there is no food (this was clearly demonstrated in concentration camps during World War II), you will discover as you read on that overeating is only partially responsible for the accumulation of excess body fat. If we do not take into account the other reasons for accumulating excesses, we will never find a way to solve it.

4. Excess Body Fat Due to Eating Between Meals

Many people believe that snacking favors fat accumulation, and recommend that you eat only three meals a day.

Martin Kathan explains in his book *Beyond Diet* the effects of different eating patterns on body fat accumulation:

1. A group of test subjects was permitted to eat only during two hours a day, rather than spreading their meals throughout the day as had been their custom. They ended up with 30% more fat.

2. Another group was kept on intermittent fasts (for 24 hours once a week). This increased their capacity to transform food into fat, and so an increase in body fat was also observed among them.

3. When both test groups were examined, it was found that their alimentary canals had increased in size and weight.

4. Part of what we eat is transformed into heat, a process known as thermogenesis. This process is more efficient in the morning and diminishes as the day advances. We are programmed to eat more in the morning and to curtail consumption by night. Therefore, those who do not have breakfast and eat most of their food in the afternoon or evening encourage the accumulation of body fat.

5. The ability to transform food into heat increases when you eat many times a day and each new intake accelerates the general function of the body (the basal metabolism). Those who eat five or more times a day usually weigh less than those who have three or fewer meals per day.

If we carefully analyze these studies, we may conclude that fasting promotes the accumulation of excess body fat. Frequent fasting, far from resolving the problem, eventually causes greater fat accumulation. To rid yourself of excess body fat, you must learn to eat many times a day.

The quantity of food is not as important as the way in which you eat it.

5. Excess Body Fat Due to Heredity

Many people believe that being overweight is the result of an "evil" gene inherited from their parents which has altered their metabolism. But scientists who have analyzed this factor report contradictory results. While some find a genetic connection between overweight parents and overweight children, others attribute the connection to the eating patterns developed by the family.

An interesting study found that children born from obese mothers that were adopted to thin families had the same tendency to accumulate excess body fat as their obese biological mothers. No relationship was found with the weight of the biological fathers. This suggests that the tendency to accumulate fat is transmitted during pregnancy by mechanisms that have nothing to do with genetics: It has also been reported that when a baby is malnourished in the womb, this increases the likelihood that he will develop abdominal obesity in adulthood (after age 30), even when the biological mother is not overweight.

This situation is very common in underdeveloped countries, but it is also found in pregnant women of developed countries who purposefully reduce their food intake in order to avoid gaining excess body fat during pregnancy. Not only do they ruin their own metabolism and risk gaining weight later themselves, but they also doom their children to become obese adults. Unfortunately this was not known in the decades of the 50's through 80's and many pregnant women went on diet without knowing how much damage they were generating in their children. This is just one of many ways in which diets have converted America into a Land of the Fat.

In Canada, Claude Bouchan carried out studies on genetically identical twins. He found a tendency to gain excess fat due to genetic factors, but the same study on non-identical twins reported different results. He concluded that a genetic tendency does not explain the high incidence of excess body fat in the Canadian population.

The firmest evidence against the theory that excess body weight is due primarily to heredity is found in the analysis of emigrant populations. Japanese, who traditionally have very little excess fat, gain weight when they move to the United States. Once they leave their native country, they have the same probability of gaining excess weight as native-born Americans.

An obesity gene was recently discovered, responsible for regulating the body's production of a protein called leptin. Yet this gene is found in thin people as well as overweight people. We are all born with the necessary genes to develop excess body fat. It is just a matter of applying improper eating habits and any human body will defend itself by accumulating fat.

THE REAL REASON

You see, alterations to the normal human metabolism do exist, but they are attributable to eating habits more than to genetics. Studies have shown that overweight people have a normal basal metabolism as long as they don't go on a diet. Bad eating habits do not destroy the normal functions of the body, but they do alter them. For instance, bad eating habits do not eliminate the body's ability to transform excess food into heat, but they do reduce it.

According to genetic studies, the ability to accumulate excess body fat is a biological weapon for survival, and not a curse for the fashion-conscious. When food intake is restricted, the body responds to this scarcity of food by increasing its tendency to store fat.

The United States has carried out periodic surveys of its general population, known as NHANES (National Health and Nutrition Examination Survey). The most recent NHANES showed an increase in the number of obese Americans, from 15% of the population in 1980 to 27% in 1999. It has been calculated that if this tendency persists, by the year 2050, 90% of the American population will be overweight and/or obese.

According to a telephonic interview, at any given moment, 36% of the American population is dieting to try to lose weight. In 1985, when I first came to the conclusion that diets make you fat, I predicted that if Americans continued with the yo-yo syndrome, by the 22nd century almost all would be overweight. Unfortunately, I miscalculated. I underestimated the problem. If we do not learn to eat to lose weight, excess body fat will quickly become the most serious health problem in the country and the same is true for other developed countries.

This increasing level of obesity is strong evidence against the theory that excess body fat is the result of genetic factors and strong evidence in favor of the theory that the accumulation of excess body fat is a mechanism for survival triggered by dieting.

Even the strongest defenders of the theory that excess body fat is due to heredity agree that a sensible diet can reduce this tendency. Fortunately for those who are overweight, the external environment is more important than genetic factors in gaining and maintaining excess body fat.

There is a real hereditary tendency to gain weight, but it can be countered in an efficient way with a sufficient and balanced diet.

6. Excess Body Fat Due to Emotional Factors

No scientific study has demonstrated any special personality trait that favors obesity. The same percentages of thin and overweight people are depressed, passive, neurotic, obsessive, etc.

Nevertheless, the way emotional conflict is handled can favor the accumulation of body fat. Acute stress which is not quickly solved will develop into chronic stress, and this, in turn, may lead to the accumulation of body fat. The relationship between stress and obesity is a complex one, and it is very important that we study it in detail.

EXCESS BODY FAT AND STRESS

Stress, in scientific terms, is an adaptation response of a living organism to external stimuli. Bacteria, viruses, and fish, as well as human beings, experience stressing events. For example, bacteria will be stressed when facing a chemical agent (an antibiotic). As organisms become more complex, stress takes different forms. The chase of a tiger after a gazelle brings stress to both.

Human beings have carried stress to an even more complicated level. If we face a dangerous event, such as almost being run over by a car, we experience an organic response to stress at that moment and at every other moment that we remember the incident. Our ability to generate stress through our thoughts explains how stress can damage our body. We stimulate defense mechanisms just by thinking of a stressful event. Simply watching an exciting movie produces metabolic reactions.

That is why the definition of stressing events varies enormously in human beings. What some consider dangerous may be highly pleasurable to others. Driving a car at high speed may be very exciting for some but nerve-wracking for others.

Our organic response to stress is also different according to the time we are exposed to it. Stress can be either acute or chronic.

Acute stress causes the body to release a series of substances, including adrenaline and cortisone. Adrenaline eliminates body fat directly through mobilization (converting fat to energy for use by the muscles) and indirectly by increasing the basal metabolism. It also reduces appetite. Consequently, acute stress results in weight loss. This is a very unpleasant but effective way of eliminating excess fat and muscle.

On the other hand, during **chronic stress**, excess adrenaline production stops and cortisone, which favors fat accumulation, continues to be secreted. Even so, chronic stress will produce excess fat only when associated with other events.

A natural defense mechanism against acute stress is the liberation of endorphins in the brain. These substances produce feelings of pleasure and are extraordinary for controlling pain. Pleasure generated by endorphins makes stress more tolerable. This response is automatic, and there is nothing that we can or should do to avoid it.

When enduring chronic stress, we must look for ways to free more endorphins to help us bear those unpleasant sensations associated with this chronic stress.

There are many events that liberate endorphins and generate pleasure; physical activity, sexual activity, eating, taking alcoholic beverages, and even abstract stimuli such as hearing music, reading and having pleasant thoughts.

Depending on the way you obtain extra endorphins during chronic stress, you can gain or lose body fat. Pleasure obtained through music, work, exercise, and sexual activity obviously does not lead to excess body fat. But to obtain pleasure exclusively through the consumption of fat does lead to excess body fat.

It has been shown through multiple studies that the food group which frees the most endorphins (the tastiest one) is fat. When chronically stressed, we develop a greater urge for chocolates and a lesser desire for lettuce and carrots. Bear in mind that this is the normal biological response of thin people as well as overweight people.

Someone subjected to chronic stress can easily reduce unpleasant sensations by eating fried chicken, doughnuts, pastry, and any food that is fried. If this (managing chronic stress through excessive fat consumption) is maintained for a long enough time, excess body fat will appear.

On the other hand, acute stress can also generate obesity, especially if our body is already malnourished. Remember that acute stress reduces appetite and that food restriction increases the ability to accumulate fat in a body that is already poorly nourished. Then, if acute stress becomes chronic and we manage it by eating high-fat foods, gaining weight is inevitable.

STRESSING EVENTS

This complicated situation gets even more complicated when we study what triggers stress. Being late for work can be extremely stressing for some, while others can take it very calmly. If you spend the rest of the day agonizing over the fact that you were late, you are encouraging the accumulation of excess body fat.

Stress in itself does not cause excess body weight, but stubbornly re-experiencing the stressing events again and again in our minds undoubtedly can. Whether stress causes weight gain depends on our way of handling life.

Conflicts will lead to excess body fat only if we allow them to alter our emotional stability and manage them by consuming excessive fat. To keep conflict and stress from ruining our health, we might have to change our lifestyle. Those who maintain satisfactory relationships at work and at home, enjoy daily physical activity, and derive pleasure from ordinary tasks will not need to eat fatty foods in order to handle stressing events.

7. Excess Body Fat Due to Excess Fat in the Diet

The relationship between fat in the diet and excess body fat is very important. There is no doubt that excessive fat in a diet can cause obesity.

All studies on this topic show that a direct relationship exists between fat in the diet and excess body weight. Scientific evidence in this regard is both epidemiological (when the eating habits of large populations are studied) and experimental (when controlled experiments are conducted on smaller groups of people). For instance, some experimental studies have shown that people gain excess fat very quickly when adding 80 grams of fat to their usual diet. Excessive fat consumption is definitely the prime villain in this story.

The human body has a series of defenses to protect us from consuming excessive amounts of carbohydrates (sugars). Occasional excess amounts of sugar are burned with ease. When a diet is very high in sugar, the sensation of flavor decreases, and thus, with time, over consumption is usually curtailed. Current medical studies have stated that high-sugar diets, although harmful for the body, are not directly related to excess body weight.

Dietary fat, on the other hand, produces the opposite effect. A high-fat diet will always be tastier, and therefore make us eat more than we need. Excessive fat consumption is not curtailed with time, and, as will be explained later on, dietary fat is easily stored in the body.

The preference for fat can be demonstrated from the day we are born and will continue for the rest of our lives, whether we are thin or not. This natural desire is intended to help us survive in situations where food is not always available. Ingested fat passes to the waist, and is stored there, to be used when needed, but only after weeks of food deprivation.

Our food usually contains large quantities of fat, and we almost always add more when preparing it.

The primitive and spontaneous craving for fat in our meals leads to excessive consumption, and consequently fat is accumulated in the body. That is why six out of ten American adults are overweight. If bad eating habits also exist (fear of food, fasting, constant dieting, etc.), obesity (very high levels of excess body fat) appears. That is why three out of six of those who are overweight become obese.

What happens if we consciously and severely limit the fat in our diet? The negative effects can range from dry skin to damage to our immune systems. Perhaps you would be willing to tolerate these negative consequences in order to achieve a thin body. But there is one more negative effect that you might not expect; diets very low in fat lead to more accumulation of body fat.

Fat is a necessary element of our diet. Depending on where you live, more or less is required. In tropical zones, 25% to 30% of calories from fat in your diet are usually enough. In higher latitudes, the requirement can increase to 35%. Eskimos who lived under primitive conditions had diets with more than 50% fat.

Diets very low in fat (less than 20% of total calories) may trigger survival mechanisms. But even if survival mechanisms are activated, excess body fat will not appear as long as the diet continues to contain less than 20% fat. Unfortunately, a body with an activated survival mechanism will accumulate excess body fat as soon as even small quantities of extra fat are added to the diet.

I will explain this in another way. Those who never diet may include up to 40% fat in their menu and remain slender. But if they restrict their fat intake to less that 20% of total calories for a long enough time, they can activate the starvation mode. Once the starvation mode is activated, the fat that they were accustomed to eat will now accumulate around their waist.

We're damned when excess fat exists in our diets, but even more damned when fat is drastically reduced.

This phenomenon has been observed in two different cultures.

People in rural Mexico usually eat a diet that is very low in fats (around 20%, according to Mexico's National Institute of Nutrition). When they migrate to the United States and start eating a normal fat or high-fat diet, they accumulate excess fat more quickly than the general American population. Worse still, fat is deposited around the waist, thus increasing the frequency of diabetes.

In Japan, where excess body fat was seldom a problem, people were used to eating a diet in which 20% of total calories came from fat. Now that they have been invaded by America's fast food and high-fat restaurants, excess body fat is becoming a significant problem.

The Chinese obtain less than 20% of their calories from fat and they eat from 2,500 to 3,000 calories per day. This is roughly 500 more calories than Americans, and yet excess weight is very rare in China. If the Chinese adopt a Western diet that is high in fat (around 40%), they will certainly face an epidemic of excess body fat greater than that in America.

When I came to understand that excess body fat was generated by the relative amount of fat in the diet rather than the absolute amount, I predicted these events years before they were reported.

The discovery that low-fat diets as well as high-fat diets increased the risk of developing excess body weight led researchers to investigate what minimum amount of fat were needed in a diet and which fats were best for our bodies.

A normal balanced diet should include approximately one gram of fat per day for every two pounds of ideal body weight. Even the strictest weight-loss diets should include small quantities of fat. Most experts recommend at least 40 grams per day for males and 20 grams per day for females.

Scientists have also reported that certain dietary fats may help you lose weight. Let me explain.

Just as there are different types of sugars, so there are different types of fats, and the body handles them differently. Fats have been classified as saturated, monounsaturated, and polyunsaturated. Saturated fats are found in warm-blooded animals, as well as certain vegetables such as coconut oil.

Monounsaturated fats are mainly found in olive oil and nuts. Polyunsaturated fats are obtained from seeds, such as corn and sunflowers, and are usually used for cooking. Many marine species also contain polyunsaturated fats. Fat that is found in a liquid state at room temperature is sure to contain large quantities of monounsaturated or polyunsaturated fats.

Although controversy exists, it seems that a diet high in saturated fats may cause severe problems, including cancer and excess body fat.

The book *The Paleolithic Prescription*, written by S. Boyd Eaton, makes an interesting analysis of food ingested by our ancestors more than 10,000 years ago. Eaton concludes that human beings ate large quantities of wild animal protein, but he points out that fat content of wild animals scarcely reached 1% (similar to the levels found today in fish and shellfish). The total quantity of saturated fat ingested thousands of years ago was minimal compared to the amount of polyunsaturated fat our ancestors obtained through vegetables.

Today, the domesticated animals we eat contain large quantities of fat. In fact, the minimum fat content is 20%–which represents a 2000% increase in the amount of animal fat in the daily diet. We have not had enough time, in evolutionary terms, to adapt to such an impressive increase in this substance in our diet. Imagine what would happen if our sugar or protein consumption was increased by that amount.

Apparently most useful fats are obtained from the vegetable kingdom. Not only do they help in cell construction (a third of cell membranes and nearly 80% of our brains are made of fat), but they may also help us stay slender. This discovery has been vital in the treatment of excess body fat. A summary of studies on vegetable fats and their benefits can be found in the book *Beyond Pritikin* written by Ann Louise Gittleman.

Of special interest is gamma linoleic acid, which is believed may increase the body's ability to eliminate excess fat. According to Gittleman, this is a fat that burns fat. This substance is found in sunflower and corn oil, as well as almonds, peanuts, pistachios, and other nuts.

Then why are we not all thin if it we usually cook with vegetable oils and almost everyone loves pistachios and nuts? According to Gittleman, the reason is that when gamma linoleic acid is heated, it loses its power to eliminate fat and becomes itself fattening. Heated vegetable oils, if taken in excessive quantities, may cause excess body fat. We should eat nuts raw and keep vegetable oil in the refrigerator to use as a dressing and not for cooking as is our custom.

When polyunsaturated fats are heated or, worse still, heated several times (refried), free radicals are generated. Some investigators consider that this custom, besides favoring excess body fat, increases the frequency of cancer in the large intestine and the mammary and prostate glands and favors the development of atherosclerosis (hardening of the arteries).

If you wish to fry a food, use a monounsaturated fat such as olive oil, since this fat is very stable under high, sustained temperatures. Communities that surround the Mediterranean Sea cook with olive oil, and it is believed that this custom diminishes the risk of heart attacks, as well as the risk of cancer in different parts of the body.

The high consumption of saturated fats and the heating of polyunsaturated fats, combined with poor eating habits (constant dieting, eating with fear, skipping meals, or drastically reducing the consumption of any food group), favors the accumulation of excess body fat.

Those who wish to stay thin should cook with monounsaturated fats and reduce the amount of saturated fats and heated polyunsaturated fats in their diets. Recently, it has been demonstrated that adding conjugated linoleic acid to a diet may help people lose weight and keep it from coming back.

Attention has been drawn to vegetable oils that are hardened when combined with hydrogen. They are called trans-fatty acids and are found in foods such as vegetable shortening, some margarine, crackers, candies, baked goods, cookies, snack foods, fried foods, salad dressings, and many other processed foods.

There is a direct, proven relationship between diets high in trans-fatty acids and high LDL (low density lipoprotein) cholesterol levels, which increase the risk of coronary heart disease.

How can we know that a product contains trans-fatty acids? If the ingredient list includes the words "shortening," "partially hydrogenated vegetable oil," or "hydrogenated vegetable oil," the food contains trans-fat. Because ingredients are listed in descending order of predominance, smaller amounts are present when this ingredient is close to the end of the list. The US Food and Drug Administration (FDA) has instructed food manufacturers to add trans-fatty acid content to the "Nutrition Information" on their products' labels. It is hoped that this will reduce the amount of trans-fatty acids that we eat. Until then, it is advisable that you steer clear of products containing the ingredients mentioned above.

8. Excess Body Fat and Carbohydrates

Excess body fat is not caused by eating a high-carbohydrate diet. Contrary to popular belief, foods with high sugar content, such as bread, rice, beans, potatoes, pasta, and bananas, are necessary to control excess weight.

Continuous, excessive consumption of refined sugars can result in excess body fat, but only if they are consumed in high quantities. There is generally no natural tendency to eat more sugars than required, and with time sugar over consumption is usually and spontaneously curtailed, preventing excessive consumption.

In the following pages, recent studies related to this subject will be presented.

SUGARS AND EXCESS BODY FAT

There is a widespread and erroneous belief that carbohydrates (sugars) in the diet are responsible for excess body fat. Because of this idea, the overweight are often advised to avoid traditional dishes based on wheat products such as pasta and bread. Those who believe that eating great quantities of bread and pasta make you fat will be amazed to find that this is false.

For years, it was believed that sugars caused obesity, and therefore many diets that reduced their consumption were created. However, in the 1980s, an opposite method became very popular, and diets were developed that attempted to eliminate body fat through high sugar consumption.

Unfortunately, by the end of the century, this healthy tendency gave way to the old low-carb diets. Why? Because previous high-carbohydrate diets recommended 20% or less fat, and, as I previously stated, this can result in greater obesity in the long run when even small amounts of extra fat are added to the diet.

Where did the idea of a high-carb weight loss diet come from? We owe this to an engineer who was told he had only a few days of life remaining because his arteries were clogged. He studied the habits of primitive cultures, whose members typically have normal arteries. In 1974, Nathan Pritikin published his book *Live Longer Now*, which analyzed eating habits of Tarahumaras of Mexico and the Bantus of Africa. He concluded that these tribe's people have a low incidence of atherosclerosis (clogged arteries and other blood vessels) because of the special way they eat. According to Pritikin, in order to maintain excellent health and to diminish atherosclerosis, we should eat sufficient quantities of complex carbohydrates and reduce or even eliminate fat consumption.

Pritikin's recommendations gained great acceptance, since people could lose excess fat by eating food that tradition said would generate excess body fat. The studies done by Pritikin were so important that at present it is very rare to find scientific publications that attribute excess body fat exclusively to carbohydrates.

Pritikin lived much longer than his doctors had predicted, and when he died, his autopsy showed that atherosclerosis had receded. Unfortunately Dr. Atkins, who all his life promoted low-carbohydrate, high-fat diets, did not have an autopsy, and we will never know if his program generated or protected him from atherosclerosis.

How do you lose weight through eating beans, pasta, bread, and other foods that are reduced or prohibited in many diets? To understand why these programs work, we will study the way the body handles sugars.

SUGARS AND DIGESTION

Before we absorb and utilize what we eat, we must first digest it. Not all food groups are digested with the same ease. The most difficult is protein. Sugars are also difficult to digest, especially if they are eaten as beans, potatoes, and bread (complex carbohydrates). Which nutrients are digested most easily, passing almost intact into our bodies? Dietary fat.

The more difficult the digestion, the higher the amount of energy needed for digestion; therefore not everything that we swallow is accounted for as total caloric intake.

When we eat 100 grapes, the caloric equivalent of 23 grapes are used to obtain sufficient energy for their digestion. It follows that only 77 will be ultimately stored by the body. When we eat 100 grams of fat, only three are burned in the process of digestion; the remainder is easily stored, and fat is accumulated in the body.

Did you have trouble following this explanation? There is no reason to despair, since these findings are very easy to apply. Let's see what benefits we can obtain from all of this information.

Those who eat large quantities of unrefined sugars will seldom develop excess body fat since the body uses a great deal of energy in the process of digestion. Those who prefer a high-fat diet easily accumulate fat, since almost all of it ends up being absorbed by the body. One study demonstrated that adding 80 grams of fat (equivalent to 720 calories) to a normal diet resulted in a rapid weight gain. When the same amount of calories was added in the form of protein and sugar, no weight gain was observed.

Acheson administered 500 grams of glucose (equivalent to the amount of sugar found in 35 slices of bread or 13 cups of cooked spaghetti) to obese subjects, and found that fat was not accumulated during the following nine hours.

This explains why there is no relationship between how much you eat and how much you weigh and why there is a direct link between the quantity of fat in a diet and excess body fat.

How do we benefit from these studies? We learn that if we are going to overeat, it is preferable to select complex carbohydrates and/or protein in order to reduce the risk of generating excess body fat.

COMPLEX CARBOHYDRATES AND EXCESS BODY FAT

Sugars are present in nature in many forms: one-molecule sugars (monosaccharides), two-molecule sugars (disaccharides), and multiple-molecule sugars (polysaccharides). Monosaccharides and disaccharides are also called simple carbohydrates. Polysaccharides (many-bonded molecules) are known as complex carbohydrates.

The body digests complex carbohydrates with great difficulty and absorbs them very slowly; this is of great benefit since it reduces the risk of developing excess body fat.

When we include small amounts of complex carbohydrates and high quantities of fat in our diet, it is very difficult to feel full, and excess dietary fat is easily stored in the body! When we increase the amount of complex carbohydrates, the opposite reaction occurs. Those who include great quantities of complex carbohydrates in their diets will easily feel full and therefore will eat less excess fat.

Dietary fiber, which is also a complex carbohydrate, has two beneficial actions; it first generates a greater sensation of satiety, thus reducing the total caloric intake, and second, it interferes with the body's ability to absorb fat.

All complex carbohydrates, such as pasta, cereals, beans, lentils, and potatoes, are considered ideal foods in the new methods of reducing body fat.

THE GLYCEMIC INDEX AND EXCESS BODY FAT

Not all sugars (carbohydrates) are absorbed by the body at the same speed. Some are absorbed very quickly, while others take a longer time to be digested and absorbed. These time differences have been organized in a chart labeled the Glycemic Index. A higher number on this index means that a sugar is absorbed more quickly, and a lower number is given to sugars that are absorbed more slowly. The standard of reference for absorption is white bread.

Many studies have been carried out with diets that contain slowly absorbed carbohydrates, and they have reported that even when taken ad libitum (that is to say, the tested subjects eat as much as they wanted until they could not eat any more); people still lost weight and inches. Even more important is that these programs protect the body from cancer and heart attacks.

Here is a list of food with high carbohydrate content and a medium or low glycemic index:

> **Baked products**: apple muffins, banana cake, chocolate cake, pound cake, sponge cake, and white cake.

- **Beverages**: apple juice, carrot juice, grapefruit juice (unsweetened), fresh fruit juice, pineapple juice (unsweetened), and tomato juice (no sugar added).

- **Breads**: barley bread, buckwheat bread, corn tortillas, fruit bread, oat bran bread, whole grain wheat bread, and wheat tortillas.

- **Breakfast cereals**: Cereals made of bran and oat bran.

- **Cereal grains**: brown rice.

- **Dairy products and alternatives**: ice cream, whole milk, skim milk, pudding, soy milk, and yogurt.

- **Fruits**: apples, bananas, cherries, grapefruit, grapes, kiwis, mangoes, peaches, pears, plums, and strawberries.

- **Legumes**: black beans, butter beans, chickpeas, kidney beans, lentils, navy beans, peas, pinto beans, Romano beans, soybeans, small red beans and split peas.

- **Pasta and noodles**: capellini, fettuccine, gnocchi, instant noodles, linguine, macaroni, ravioli, and spaghetti.

- **Snack foods**: cashew nuts, M&M peanuts, Nutella, nuts, roasted almonds, peanut butter, and peanuts.

- **Vegetables**: carrots, green peas, nopal (edible cactus), sweet corn, and yams.

Were you surprised to find such items as ice cream and sponge cake in the list? When you mix sugar with protein and/or fat, that sugar is absorbed more slowly. This also happens with vinegar and lemon juice, which can reduce the glycemic index by 20 to 40%. This is why I recommend that, whenever possible, you accompany any fruit, fruit juice, or soft drink with nuts and that you add vinegar to your salads and lemon juice to any plate.

Several years ago, anchormen and reporters of an important radio station in Mexico City heard me state that if you were going to have a soft drink, you should make sure that it contained sugar and that you combined it with nuts. They all decided to try out this approach and lost several inches from their waists. From that reason, they named my program "the Coca-Cola diet."

I definitely do not recommend that soft drinks be used as a base for any diet, since many investigators believe that an increase in the intake of high fructose (the type of sugar that soft drinks use) is associated with excess body fat. But then again, if you are going to have a soft drink, accompany it with meals that contain protein and/or fats, such as nuts, hamburgers, or pizzas.

George Bray (whom I personally consider the father of the modern-day study of excess body fat) called attention to the fact that after 1980, when high-fructose corn syrup began to be used in soft drinks and many other foods, the percentage of the population that was overweight doubled. Whether this was due to dieting pregnant mothers of the 1960s and 70s, the excessively low-fat diets of the 1980s, a direct effect of these sugars or a combination of all these factors is not clear. But just to be on the safe side, steer away from these sugars.

Besides, there are so many other great low-glycemic options that I am sure you will find tasty options that will help you avoid malnutrition and under-nutrition.

It is not known whether pastry gives protection to the heart, since the low-glycemic index diets studied have relied heavily on fruits, whole grain cereals, and legumes, not pastry. Pastry probably doesn't help. This is the reason why I added pastry until the sixth week of the Bolio System.

As a rule of thumb, non-processed complex carbohydrates such as pears, bananas, apples, and grapefruit are absorbed more slowly by the body. This also happens with whole grain cereals; with nuts, pastry, and ice cream; and with legumes. The Bolio System relies heavily on these food groups.

I have described only a few of the many studies carried out on carbohydrates. The easiest way to convince you that the reported studies are correct is by convincing you to eat carbohydrates so you can see for yourself that you lose weight and inches!

9. Summary: the Causes of Excess Body Fat

For decades, excess body fat was considered to be an aesthetic inconvenience and not a health problem. That is, people wanted to lose weight because excess body fat looked ugly rather than because it was dangerous to their health. Therefore, serious research was seldom carried out. In the absence of scientific knowledge, anyone could invent his own theory of what caused excess body fat and, even worse, his own way of treating it.

Now, however, the causes of excess body fat have been identified through solid scientific research. Although many unknown variables still exist, the culprit has been defined with precision, and we can prepare sensible strategies to eliminate it. Those who sincerely want to solve the problem of excess body fat will do well to rid their minds of the old myths and rely on science.

There are four main causes of excess body fat:

1. **Malnutrition, resulting in increased metabolic efficiency or starvation mode** (see chapter one)
2. **Fasting** (see chapter four)
3. **Chronic uncontrolled stress** (see chapter six)
4. **Overeating with predominance of dietary fat** (see chapter seven)

Unfortunately, weight loss programs have paid major attention to the overeating phenomenon. Even when overeating will indeed make you fat, the other three causes play a much greater role in accumulation of excess body fat.

In the Bolio System, attention is focused on what is not eaten instead of what is overeaten. When you pay attention to what you HAVE TO EAT to be nourished and healthy, the overeating phenomenon will be spontaneously controlled.

Focus your attention on what you must eat. This is the logical way to solve this problem.

What can we say about the traditional approach to treating excess body fat?

First of all, don't be deceived by the short-term effects of diets. It is true that you lose weight, but this reaction is transitory, and sooner or later the weight will always come back. More importantly, the initial weight reduction is caused by the loss of muscle and liquids, not fat.

Those with excess body fat will be confronted with many programs that claim to help them reduce body fat. However, objective long-term results are never achieved when they are based on the erroneous belief that you only have to stop eating to solve the problem. People will lose weight, only to gain it back again and again. Fat is not lost; it is just temporarily shifted. People on a diet are the only true losers in this endless "yo-yo" game.

How can excess body fat be treated in such a manner that permanent fat loss is obtained? Through a diet that is not only sufficient, but also balanced according to the recommendations of all the major medical associations.

PART TWO
REDUCING EXCESS BODY FAT

10. The Diet-Disaster Phenomenon

Since the Bolio System allows and even promotes the ingestion of all food groups such as pastry, hamburgers, etc., it is very important that you recognize and define the *Diet-Disaster Phenomenon* before you begin. Let me explain:

In my clinical practice I stumbled over what I considered was as a very bizarre conduct: when adding pastry and candy to many of my patient's diets, they would make a spectacularly disordered program. No matter what balanced menu they received, they would always show disastrous adherence.

The only way I could convince them to return to an orderly program was to apply menus that *felt* like very strict diets. There are many ways in which you can elaborate high calorie diets that *seem* to be a very strict weight loss plan. With these types of meals, patients would return to a disciplined attitude.

When given menus that were truly bland and monotonous, they would apply themselves with great joy and discipline.

At first I thought that this was due to a masochistic attitude where patients could only accept self punishment for being overweight. I now believe the explanation has nothing to do with self punishment:

Many people have been on severely strict diets during so much time, that they only live two events in their lives; the desperation of being overweight with the subsequent application of drastic weight reduction programs, or the total loss of control after months of dieting with the subsequent application of a disastrously disorderly diet. Once they fall into desperation again, they repeat the cycle.

This is an incredible programming that even goes against primitive eating patterns. That is to say, they are either on *DIET* and applying recommendations with great discipline, or they are on *DISASTER* and will precisely do that: follow totally aberrant eating patterns. They are never eating in a normal way.

Too many people who apply my System will fail when adding variety to their menu, since it works as a trigger for the appearance of this disastrous pattern. I call this the *Diet-Disaster Phenomenon*.

This is why the first four weeks of the Bolio System are very limited in variety but free in caloric intake. They do not need to be so, for a balanced diet that includes pastry and any other food group will reduce body fat. However, because of the *Diet-Disaster Phenomenon* many will need to apply weeks one through four before advancing to menus that have greater variety.

How do you know if you are a prisoner of the *Diet-Disaster Phenomenon?*

If you start with weeks five through seven and find yourself being very disorderly in its application, then it is very probable that you have programmed yourself to either be on diet or on disaster. Therefore, you should go back to recommendations marked from weeks one to four, where the program *looks like a diet*.

Remember that the Bolio System has nothing to do with calories, and that you must always eat enough to be satiated al day long. This free caloric intake is obtained through the ingestion of the shakes marked in the Recovery Phase.

In the Recovery Phase (Weeks One and Two) shakes and protein supplements are the basic sustention. You can use these elements in any other moment of the program, since they will help you hike up the calories in an orderly fashion that *also looks like a diet*. Said another way, you will be eating great quantities of calories in a program that feels very strict.

I will repeat this one more time; even though the first four weeks of the program do in fact consist of a very strict program, they have no relationship with calorie restriction.

They are there to help those with the *Diet-Disaster Phenomenon*.

The shakes of the Recovery Phase are really fantastic since you can take as many as you want and still quickly lose excess fat, but can you use shakes and protein supplements as your basic meal plan? The answer is: definitely no.

Recent research has suggested that a healthy diet must necessarily include fruits, vegetables, whole grain cereals, nuts, seed, etc. The use of vitamin and protein supplements alone cannot be considered a healthy diet since they do not seem to confer protection against chronic diseases.

As a matter of fact, you will be applying these recommendations because you have concluded that, indeed, EATING MAKES YOU SKINNY. And the word eating includes all food groups; even the ones that may make you gain excess weight.

When are you going to learn to eat all food groups if you never add them to your life?

It's like trying to learn to ride a bike without a bike, or to swim without water. Sure, it's frightening to get on a bike or jump in the water, but there is no other way to learn. You can start with training wheels and flotation devices (weeks one to four) and later advance to a regular bike and swimming freely in a pool (weeks five through seven). Once you feel confident, you can advance to riding your bike in the mountains or swimming in the ocean (weeks eight and nine).

Are there people that can jump on a bike and ride it like an expert? Can someone solve his excess fat just by reading the book and not applying a structured program? Probably so, but I still haven't met that person yet. As a matter of fact, I have had the opportunity of meeting extremely brilliant and creative people who understood and believed in my theory, but continued to be fat because they did not apply a structured program. If you do obtain a slender and healthy body just by intuition, please let me know.

Therefore, I definitely do not recommend that you start with week nine which is the hardest one to apply in a balanced manner. It is better that you leave it for the moment you have learned to fill your body with sufficient nutritious and balanced meals at all times.

Now that you have a broad outline of what to expect from the program, let's get more specific as to what and how to do what is right to eat to be skinny.

11. Walking: the Perfect Exercise

Lack of exercise does not cause excess body fat, and programmed physical activity does not help us eliminate it. Inappropriate physical activity can even favor greater fat accumulation.

Then is it a myth that exercise helps you eliminate excess fat?

Just as with fats and sugars, our body reacts in a special way to different types of physical activity, and the response is directly related to its intensity. Intense physical activity is of little use in eliminating excess body fat. Even worse, when combined with an unbalanced diet, it can increase abdominal fat.

Those who spend their life "sweating it out" achieve only very small reductions in body fat. Many even quit exercising when they realize that it is slowly making their problem worse.

However, there is one physical activity that helps to significantly reduce body fat, converting fat into energy. What is this remarkable breakthrough exercise? It is walking. Yes, walking. Its benefits start only 15 minutes after the activity has begun and reach their maximum effect after only 30 minutes.

No technique, diet, or medication known to date generates such a quick response. Walking also reduces more fat than any other physical activity per unit of time. If you have little time to dedicate to exercise, walk. After only 15 minutes of starting to walk, you are already achieving benefits. If you can increase the time to 30 or 45 minutes, it is much better.

Many overweight people are convinced that the more intense the exercise, the more fat they will burn off. This is false. Intense physical activity burns sugar (glucose), not fat (triglycerides). When you run 100 yards at maximum speed, your body burns 100% glucose and 0% triglycerides. Walking is the activity that burns the most fat per unit of time (60% triglycerides and 40% glucose). Intense exercise limits the possibility of reducing fat around the waist.

If you are interested in being the fastest overweight person in your neighborhood, run. If you want to solve your weight problem, walk.

It has been demonstrated that overweight people use the same energy when walking that thin individuals use when running. Excess weight generates a higher consumption of calories in any type of physical activity.

Have great respect for the simple act of walking, since it is an extraordinary activity.

Walking is classified as an aerobic exercise, just like swimming, bicycle riding, and aerobics.

It will help improve muscle tone and muscle strength, thus avoiding developing a flabby body during weight-reduction programs. Even more importantly, it will greatly improve your cardiovascular and respiratory systems. As walking is prolonged, fat reserves are burned up and muscles are strengthened through repetitive movement.

Besides being a useful weight-loss tool, walking can be a pleasant activity that reduces stress and raises morale. Exercise increases self-esteem, reduces depression, and helps eliminate the tensions and stresses of daily life.

If you have decided to walk, it is important that you reap all of its benefits.

What is the ideal time to walk? Maximum benefit is obtained if you walk shortly after waking up in the morning and 15 minutes after eating the heaviest meal of the day. Those who have difficulty managing carbohydrates, such as the metabolic syndrome and diabetes, will find greater benefit when walking before their largest meal. But do not turn your life upside down to exercise at an ideal time. A better recommendation is to walk when you can most enjoy it.

Many housewives say that they normally walk more than two hours a day during their usual activities. This is quite true, but intermittent walking is less efficient in burning fat, since you must maintain continuous activity for at least 15 minutes in order to obtain the direct mobilization of body fat.

The amount of time that you walk is also important: 150 minutes a week is considered the minimum that will help you reduce incidence of chronic disease. For an evident loss of body fat, at least 200 minutes per week are needed. In my personal opinion, best results are obtained when you walk every day of the week. I also believe that it is better to have two thirty minute sessions per day than a one hour session ever 24 hours.

What if you find some other type of physical activity more enjoyable or you have already started a different exercise program? Feel free to continue doing whatever you are doing. Any aerobic activity will burn fat as long as it is moderate and does not produce pain or profuse sweating.

Pay careful attention to the intensity of your physical activity. Violent exercise enlarges your muscles and increases your strength, but it does not help you eliminate excess fat. If you enjoy cycling (either outdoors or on an indoor exercise bike), go ahead. But if you are experiencing muscle pain, fatigue, profuse sweating, or shortness of breath, you are actually inhibiting the burning of fat.

There is a simple way to determine how intense your activity should be: Subtract your age from 220, and then multiply the result by 0.6. For example, if you are 40 years old, 220 minus 40 equals 180, and 180 multiplied by 0.6 is 108. This means that your median heart rate when exercising should be 108 if you want to burn off the maximum amount of body fat.

If you start with week one or week three of the Bolio System (see part three), reduce your physical activity to a minimum. Until you learn to eat without fear, the energy (number of calories) that you receive in these weeks can be somewhat limited. Therefore, it is possible that even moderate activity will encourage accumulation of body fat. Keep in mind that, to date, there is no such thing as the "Overweight Olympics". Do not try to be become the best fat athlete in your neighborhood.

If you have been involved in intense and constant physical activity (that is, more than an hour a day, more than four times a week, for more than three months), start the Bolio System with the food prescribed for weeks four to seven plus all the shakes that you desire.

12. The Myth of the Scale

There is no greater anguish for those on a diet than stepping onto the scale. Imagine strictly adhering to a very rigid diet that causes hunger, abdominal pain, and mood swings, and then getting onto the scale, only to find that you have not only not lost weight, but you have even gained a little. Apprehension quickly turns into frustration, and frustration turns into fury as you realize that you have fallen short of your goal. This happens to more than 20% of the people who start a diet. What is worse, sooner or later it happens to all who are on a strict diet; no matter how faithfully they stick to the plan, eventually they will stop losing weight and regain some, or all, of what they have lost.

Unfortunately, for years, the medical community has erroneously insisted that overweight patients constantly monitor their weight. The story of the scale is a dark chapter in the history of humanity's attempts to deal with excess body fat. Millions around the world have been tortured (and are still being tortured) by the tyranny of the scale. There is no sense in focusing your energy only on losing weight. Turn your attention away from the scale, and concentrate instead on your body measurements.

The major problem with measuring body weight is that it has very low "specificity." The term "specificity," frequently used in medicine, refers to the ability of a study or test to diagnose an illness with precision. For example, body temperature is non-specific. Taking a patient's temperature will reveal that he has fever, but it does not tell us if he has the fever because he has an infection, has a brain hemorrhage, has developed some type of cancer, or is having an allergic reaction.

Similarly, weight is modified by many factors that have nothing to do with the loss or gain of body fat. Following are some examples:

EXAMPLE 1: A woman who is anxious to lose excess body fat decides to weigh herself daily. During her menstrual cycle, despite the fact that she has adhered strictly to her very restrictive diet, she finds to her surprise that she has gained weight. Erroneously concluding that she is gaining body fat, she restricts her diet even more despite the fact that the weight gain was due to her menstrual cycle (a true story).

EXAMPLE 2: A young woman decides to vacation in a warm climate and observes that in the first two days she has gained four pounds. She decides to start a diet while on vacation, in spite of the fact that her clothes still fit. She doesn't know that any increase in the temperature of the external environmental causes the body to retain more water. Her weight gain was due to an increase in water content, not an increase in body fat (sadly, another true story).

EXAMPLE 3: A young man decides to control his excess weight with exercise, but is disappointed when he gains weight instead of losing it. Even though his trainer explains that the weight gain is due to muscle growth, and even though his clothes start to fit better, he stops exercising in an effort to avoid gaining more weight (a true story).

EXAMPLE 4: A young woman goes to a party, where she drinks two alcoholic beverages. Two days later, she discovers she has gained three pounds and decides to start a diet to eliminate what was gained. She does not know that moderate alcohol consumption can cause a temporary retention of fluids and she has not increased her amount of body fat (a true story).

EXAMPLE 5: A woman goes to a weight-loss clinic and walks out with a bag full of "miracle pills." Over the next few days, she has to run to the bathroom every hour, and the scale shows a loss of six pounds. She pays little attention to her urgent need to urinate and continues with her treatment. She is not taking into account that her lost weight is due to water loss and not fat reduction (unfortunately, a true story).

EXAMPLE 6: A man controls his weight with a low-carbohydrate diet. On one occasion, he eats a small piece of apple pie and discovers the following day that he has gained four pounds. He incorrectly concludes, in spite of the fact that his clothes still fit, that four ounces of apple pie have been transformed into four pounds of body fat. He doesn't know that low-sugar diets dehydrate the body and that adding even small quantities of sugars can cause the body to retain water, not body fat (anyone who has been on a low-carb diet knows this story).

The scale does not define any increase or loss of body fat with precision. Worse still, it does not determine how much excess fat a body may have. When you weigh yourself, you are measuring fat, muscle, water, bone, and internal organs. You cannot know how much of your total weight consists of each element.

Excess body fat is more precisely defined by measuring circumference of abdomen and hips. The misery caused by constantly weighing yourself is not only unnecessary, but it can also give you false information on how well you are doing on a diet. If you gain muscle as you lose fat, your weight will rise. This must not be interpreted as a bad result. On the other hand, the weight loss caused by very low calorie diets is almost always due to a loss water and muscle, not fat.

As well, spontaneous weight loss is almost always an indication of a major illness, such as AIDS, diabetes, cancer, etc.

The limited information the scale provides is often not worth the emotional suffering it causes.

THE PROPER USE OF THE SCALE

Is it worthwhile to weigh yourself? If done correctly, it can serve as one of various indicators of changes taking place in your body.

Preferably, weigh yourself on a clinical scale. Use the same scale each time, since weighing yourself on many scales, with slightly different readings, will only cause confusion. Do it at the same hour of the day, for as the day advances, you always gain weight. Always do it under the same circumstances (such as, after going to the bathroom and before having a meal). Remember to weigh yourself naked or wearing only light underclothes.

And remember that even very accurate weight measurement will only tell you how much your weight has changed. It will never tell you how much fat you have lost. Therefore, the scale is of limited value in treating the problem of excess body fat, and there is little sense in using it as the sole method for measuring the effectiveness of a fat-reduction program.

A more accurate way to determine changes in body fat is "anthropometry." This is a fancy word for a simple activity: the measurement of your body with a measuring tape. If you have been measured by a tailor or seamstress, you already know what anthropometry is.

Anyone seriously interested in reducing excess fat must learn to take his body measurements. The following instructions will help you do this correctly:

HOW TO MEASURE YOURSELF

Ideally, you should take your measurements once a week, at the same hour of the day, and under similar conditions (before eating and after going to the bathroom). Use a measuring tape like those used by seamstresses. If possible, measure yourself while lying down on a firm surface.

You should be naked, or wearing only light underclothes, since thick fabrics and elastic clothes give false results. Do not adjust the tape to obtain better results. If you are honest when measuring, you will obtain an excellent indication of changes to the body. Measure your calf barefoot since high heels will modify the circumference of the calf.

If you are careless when measuring, the results will be different each time. In this case, you will erroneously conclude that you are either gaining or losing fat. Practice on multiple occasions until you are sure you are obtaining dependable results. This way you will learn to measure yourself quickly and without errors.

WHERE TO MEASURE

1. Chest: at the nipples.
2. Waist: at the belly button.
3. Buttocks: at the maximum width of the buttocks and over the pubic bone.
4. Thigh: in the groin, where the leg joins the body.
5. Calf: at the largest circumference.

You can write down the results in the following table.

Week	Chest	Waist	Buttocks	Thigh	Calf
1					
2					
3					
4					
5					
6					
7					
8					
9					
10					
11					
12					

OTHER MEASURES

Another way to monitor changes is by taking weekly pictures of your body. However, I would recommend this method only if you are comfortable with it, you have a secure way of having the photos developed and you have a secure place to keep the photos.

Finally, one of the best measures of whether you are losing excess body fat is your wardrobe. If your clothes start to fit better, you can be sure you are doing okay, even if the scale shows no changes and even if you feel that you may be getting fatter. When you have to go out and buy a smaller size, it is certain that you are losing excess body fat.

WHAT YOU FEEL WITH THIS PROGRAM

One event that puzzled me since my first treatments of obese patients was that almost all mentioned a sensation of feeling fatter, or of not losing weight.

This is quite strange since no one ever *feels* when excess body fat is being accumulated, and only through tighter clothes does anyone recognize that he indeed is getting fat. Why should anyone *feel* that they are getting thinner with traditional low calorie diets?

It is very probable that what patients *feel* when dieting is the loss of muscular mass and/or fluids, since low calorie diets will generate fat loss only after more than 10 days of dieting.

But why would patients *feel* fatter with this program, when they, in fact, are losing weight and inches? I believe that this sensation is generated by fluid retention and/or increase of muscular mass.

Therefore, if when applying the Bolio System you *feel* that you are gaining weight, or do not *feel* that you are losing anything, pay no attention to your sensations and continue with the program. As we have just stated, there are various ways (measuring tape, clothes, a photograph) in which you can demonstrate yourself that you are indeed losing excess body fat.

13. The Way You Eat Is More Important than What You Eat

I have already mentioned the negative effect of fasting meals on excess body fat. But then, what is the ideal time interval between meals? Two or three hours.

The effect of any given meal on the subsequent selection of food has been studied on many occasions. It has been discovered that what you eat now will affect what and how much you want to eat later on during the day. This effect appears as early as one hour after eating something and is most evident two to three hours later. It is known as the post-ingestive window. This effect is diminished during the rest of the day, unless, of course, you continue eating every two to three hours.

Foods that are high in sugars have a greater effect on this two-to-three-hour time span, and those with a low glycemic index and/or high fiber content have an even grater effect. Loading up with carbohydrates will not only reduce appetite in general, but will also reduce the amount of fat that you desire to eat.

As already stated, this effect is reduced after three hours, and only after 72 hours will our body again compensate for either a shortage or excess of specific nutrients.

For example, if you eat fewer fats than needed, after 72 hours your body will send the signal to add more fats than usual to your menu.

We call this sensation a "craving," and if it is clearly defined, there is no reason for it to lead to accumulation of excess body fat. Unfortunately, people with excess body fat are not wise enough to give their body exactly what it needs to stay thin. I am firmly convinced that this incapacity is based on their personal beliefs. The naturally thin tend to give in to their cravings and do not experience an emotional reaction against adding extra food to their diet since they never associate their hunger signals with excess body fat. Overweight individuals, on the other hand, have been wrongly convinced that eating makes you fat and therefore will react negatively and emotionally, refusing to listen to their cravings.

Therefore, it is prudent to use the shorter, two-to-three-hour interval between meals and allow our body to react to these internal clues.

When you eat every two to three hours, the following events will occur:

First, you will eat smaller quantities at each meal and feel satisfied. This is very important since it has been demonstrated that women over 60 years of age who eat frequent meals that have less than 400 calories per meal, will not gain excess fat. Since the Bolio System recommends seven small meals a day, in theory you could eat up to 2,800 calories per day (7 x 400 = 2,800) and not gain body fat.

And I state "in theory" because I have observed that when people eat every two to three hours a balanced diet that contains abundant legumes, fruits and vegetables, it is practically impossible to eat more than 2,200 calories.

In one unpublished study, I gave 3,000 calories per day to otherwise healthy obese women, and even though they did not lose weight, I observed an average loss of 4 cm at the waist. After the four week period, the patients had to suspend the program since they felt uncomfortable with such high quantities of food.

The second thing that will happen is that you will more clearly identify your cravings and therefore have a better opportunity to give your body what it needs. Since the Bolio System is balanced, you will be pleased to observe that after following it for two to three days, cravings will practically disappear.

The third and most important event is that when you are not exceedingly hungry, you can select healthy meals over high-fat ones. After 12 hours of fasting, it will be extremely difficult for anyone, either thin or overweight, to choose through pleasure a vegetable salad over pork chops or potato chips. Said another way, when you eat every two to three hours, it's easier to steer away from high-fat foods and enjoy meals with less fat.

Excess hunger is your worst enemy when you start the war against excess body fat. To oppose this fearsome enemy, I have discovered an amazing and extraordinary solution that will work every time you use it: **food**. It actually takes your hunger away! Isn't that incredible? Using food to take your hunger away is not only lots of fun; it is also the logical way to lose excess body fat in a permanent manner.

Last, but not least, when you eat every two to three hours, you accelerate your metabolism.

14. Choose Wisely

The information that you have read so far in this book will help you select the right foods so that you can reduce excess fat through eating from all food groups. Following are some guidelines about what kinds of choices would be wisest.

PROTEIN

In the Bolio System menus presented in section three of this book, programmed protein will fluctuate from 15% to 18% of total calories in a 24 hour span.

People in developed as well as underdeveloped countries will eat somewhere between 12% and 18% of calories from protein. The main difference between countries is not the amount of grams of protein that are eaten, but the source that is used to obtain their protein. Underdeveloped countries obtain their protein mainly from plants, while highly developed countries obtain their protein mainly from domesticated animals.

From these population studies we can conclude that protein ingestion is tightly controlled in a spontaneous manner. You might decide to carefully track all the protein that you eat, but this is really unnecessary in a sensible weight loss plan, as long as you choose protein with a low or non fat content. As a matter of fact, if you are craving food that is high in protein, then this is a clear indication that you must add it to any menu, even when it is not programmed.

From studies of the eating habits of people who live around the Mediterranean Sea, it is believed that it is wise to obtain large quantities of protein from plants and small amounts of protein from animals, while preferring fish and poultry over beef and pork. As I have stated before, reducing animal fat in the diet may not only help you stay thin, but could also reduce the incidence of heart problems and cancer. It is wise to choose lean cuts of beef and pork.

In concordance with the Mediterranean Diet, I have programmed low quantities of animal based protein in this book. Lunch will seem specially strange or different, since legumes were used as the source of vegetable protein. Perhaps this time of day will seem totally different from your usual eating habit, but it will assure a rapid and healthy loss of abdominal fat.

This is very important: you have the liberty of adding as much low fat or non fat animal or vegetable protein as you wish to any of my recommendations without affecting end results. A lean cut should have 3 grams or less of total fat per ounce of cooked serving; these include lean cuts of beef or pork, chicken breast without skin, any type of fish or shellfish, low and/or non fat milk products, egg whites and protein supplements. A fantastic place to find the fat content of many food groups is: http://www.nutritiondata.com.

All animal protein recommended in this book has a low fat content. Therefore, the weight indicated is the **minimal** quantity to eat. If you want or need more, go ahead and eat as much as you desire, since the program will not be affected by these extra quantities.

The US Food and Drug Administration recommends that you do not eat shark, swordfish, king mackerel, or tilefish because they contain high levels of mercury. Fish that are low in mercury include canned light tuna, salmon, pollock, and catfish.

Recent studies suggest that milk and soy protein favor greater fat loss and protect muscle mass from being used by the body. You can add as much of these foods as you wish, as long as you use low fat or non fat milk, milk products such as whey protein and soy protein isolate.

If you do decide to add extra protein to your program, just remember to comply with this extremely important rule: NO MATTER WHAT YOU ADD TO YOUR DAILY PROGRAM, BE IT HEALTHY OR DISASTROUS, YOU MUST STILL EAT ALL THAT IS PROGRAMMED EVEN WHEN NOT HUNGRY.

FATS

When it comes to fats, those from vegetables are more suitable for a healthy diet. First on the list are nuts and seeds, closely followed by avocado fruit, avocado oil, and olive oil that can be used for cooking. Canola and peanut oil also have good quantities of monounsaturated fats. Other vegetable oils can be used as long as they are not submitted to constant heat. Saturated fats, such as those found in butter and lard, should be used sparingly. Reduce as much as possible your intake of trans-fatty acids, which are produced when vegetable oils are hardened through hydrogen saturation (examples are margarine and non-dairy cream).

Three epidemiological studies (Nurses' Health Study, Adventists Health Study, and Physicians' Follow-up Study) report that those who eat the most nuts also tend to have the lowest body weight.

In another study, a group of free-living individuals added 320 calories of almonds (equal to 2 ounces of dry roasted almonds) to their daily diet and did not gain any weight. In my personal experience, almonds, pistachios, cashews and avocadoes give the best results when it comes to eliminating excess body fat.

Nuts in the diet may also reduce the possibility of developing type 2 diabetes and protect you from heart attacks. Nuts may also reduce LDL (the "bad" cholesterol) and hypertension.

Learn to cook without adding oil to your dishes. Food will definitely taste different, but you are investing in a healthier and thinner body. Add oil after you have cooked your meals, or preferably to your salads as dressing.

If you are going to use oil in cooking, prefer mono unsaturated oils such as olive oil.

In regards to saturated fats, don't eliminate them completely from your diet, since we do not know what will happen in the long run if you do this. Therefore, occasionally include butter and/or cream, as well as cuts of beef or pork high in fat, especially if you detect a clear craving for them...

Chocolate is a very interesting food group since it has many health benefits despite its high content of saturated fat. Therefore, not all saturated fats are bad for your body.

Desserts such as pastry have a high concentration of carbohydrates and fat. As stated before, they usually have a low glycemic index, and in theory, should be wonderful in any weight loss program.

Then of course, we have to take into account that a diet with fats submitted to high temperatures may generate, or perhaps not protect from chronic disease. I have a rule for these nutrients: take nutritious and healthy food before taking some dessert. Said another way, add them to your program as long as you eat all recommended meals, and as long as your cholesterol and triglycerides stay in a normal level. And, of course, if your speed of fat loss is slowed down when adding pastry, try to steer away from them.

Recently attention has been drawn to omega 3 fatty acids which are abundant in fish especially those found in cold waters. These acids seem to be useful in many diseases associated with inflammation. Since obesity has been recently described as having an important inflammatory component, it would seem wise to add these elements to the menu. This can be done by adding two to three fish servings per week. In this program you will add three fish portions per week.

CARBOHYDRATES

With carbohydrates, it is wise to choose from those which have a medium and/or low glycemic index, meaning that they will be absorbed slowly by the digestive tract. A list of some of these products was given in chapter eight.

However, if you do eat carbohydrates that are absorbed quickly (such as soft drinks) you can reduce their speed of absorption by accompanying them with protein and/or fat. Vinegar, as well as lemon juice, will also reduce the glycemic index.

What about fruit juice? Many epidemiologic studies have taken into account the total daily fruit servings including fresh fruit and fruit juice. They have reported that a high intake of fruits (and fruit juice) may reduce the danger of developing chronic diseases. In this book, sugars are mainly obtained from fruit, pasta, bread and legumes along with fruit juice. In my other book, *What the Naturally Skinny Do to Stay Skinny* you will find that fruit juice as well as soft drinks are used. In my experience, fruit juice has nothing to do with excess body fat as long as the program complies with the criteria of a balanced meal.

If you have a clear craving for fruit juice, go ahead and add more quantities to this program, *as long as you eat all marked meals for that day.* If this is happening on a daily basis, I recommend that you check your glucose and triglyceride levels with your doctor just to make sure they are within normal range. If he says it's OK, then continue with your free intake. It really won't affect the speed of reduction *as long as you eat all programmed meals.*

Since some investigators believe that foods with high fructose corn syrup favor fat accumulation, it is wise to stay on the safe side and prefer fruit juice over soft drinks. If you are going to have soft drinks, try taking them with nuts or seeds whenever possible.

VITAMINS, MINERALS AND FIBER

The Bolio System states that when the body does receive an insufficient amount of ANY nutrient, it will mount defense mechanisms (commonly named starvation mode) which will favor accumulation of excess body fat.

There is mounting evidence that this applies not only to macro nutrients, but to vitamins and minerals as well; insufficient amounts of certain vitamins and minerals have been linked to obesity and such is the case of calcium and vitamins C and E.

The Food and Nutrition Board of the Institute of Medicine established in 2001 the Dietary Reference Intake (DRI) which replaces previous Recommended Daily Allowance (RDA) for vitamins and minerals.

Every effort has been made so that recommendations in this book cover as much as possible these guidelines.

However, vitamin D reaches only 50 to 70% of current DRI despite the fact that fruit juice with added vitamin D is recommended. Therefore, it is wise to add 200 IU of vitamin D supplement on a daily basis.

In order to increase vitamin E content of the program I included sunflower oil which naturally contains certain amount of vitamin E. Fortunately, many companies are currently adding vitamin E to other products such as corn oil. If you decide to use a vegetable oil different from sunflower, just check the Nutrition Facts label where it should clearly mark that the product contains 20% of DRI of vitamin E for every tablespoon of product. You should preferably use this oil as salad dressing.

You should also add vitamin C supplements to the program. Even though this menu covers 300% of DRI, you will probably obtain a faster loss of excess body fat when adding 500 to 1,000 mgs extras of vitamin C to your daily menu.

These two last vitamins seem to be very important in obese middle age people who combine physical activity with their weight loss program.

It is also very important that you include at least 25 grams of soluble and non soluble fiber per day in your diet. This amount has already been programmed in the menu listed in this book.

BALANCE

These food groups should be eaten in the following proportions: You should get about 55% of you calories from carbohydrates, 15% from protein, and 30% from fat. Another way to define this is a 4:1:0.9 relationships when food is measured by weight; that is to say, for every four grams of carbohydrates, you should eat one gram of protein and 0.9 grams of fat.

Can addictive and tasty foods such as pork chops, pastry, and potato chips be included in a balanced program?

As long as what you eat is balanced, you will not accumulate excess body fat when adding these food groups to your diet. For example, two ounces of apple pie can be easily balanced with eight ounces of non-fat milk and one tsp. of brown sugar. This combination gives you 37 grams of total carbohydrates, 10 grams of total protein and 8.4 grams of total fat. This is close enough to the 4:1:0.9 relationships to keep you thin.

In weeks six and seven of the Bolio System, the mid-afternoon pastry has been balanced out with what is recommended for the rest of the day.

But keep in mind that being thin does not necessarily make you healthy, since skinny people can have high levels of cholesterol and triglycerides, and can develop heart disease, stroke, and cancer.

The ability to eat anything that you crave to become thin should not give you permission to fill yourself up with meals loaded with saturated fats, trans-fatty acids, high fructose corn sugar, and other sugars with a high glycemic index.

That is why *only* weeks six and seven indicate pastry such as cheesecake. When it comes to all those food groups that you know are not so healthy, leave them for special occasions (maybe weekends), and concentrate on giving your body what it really needs; a healthy and filling menu.

This also means that you do not have to fret over adding an occasional dish that is high in saturated fats as long as you keep eating the food groups that you know will guarantee you a healthy body.

In regards to quantities, remember that these are not important as long as you eat the foods in the proper proportions and you eat every two to three hours.

Sounds easy, right? Well, it' not, and you can demonstrate that by just taking a look around you. All these recommendations have been around for quite a while, and excess body fat persists and is even on the rise.

Solving this problem is difficult, but not impossible. Want to make it easier? Follow the Bolio System outlined in section three of this book.

15. How To Reduce or Avoid Excess Body Fat

Recent research shows that it is possible to eliminate excess body fat. But to do this requires new strategies. These include eating all kinds of food in sufficient quantities.

Studies demonstrate that there is an area of the human brain that indicates exactly what to eat, how much to eat, and when to eat it; this region is the "Center of Appetite and Satiety."

The Center of Appetite and Satiety functions properly up to age five or six. Multiple studies report how infants select perfectly balanced meals, all by themselves, just by paying attention to their body's needs.

After age six, we stop paying attention to this Center of Appetite and Satiety, and adopt eating patterns that favor fat accumulation. Unfortunately, this is so prevalent that 30% of the American population is obese, and an additional 30% has excess weight. Only 40% of the general population maintains a stable, healthy weight.

Several factors alter our ability to pay attention to the Center of Appetite and Satiety: stress (emotional tension); a lack of physical activity; excessive physical activity; sexual activity; any intensely pleasant thought; consumption of substances such as coffee, tobacco, and alcohol; and, above all, the ideas and habits that we learn about what we should or shouldn't eat. Infants, who have had excellent eating habits up to age five or six, then begin to disregard what their brains are telling them and start following inappropriate eating habits learned from family and society. At least five years of constant parental interference are required to ruin our extraordinary ability to eat in a well-balanced manner just by paying attention to our biological needs.

There is no reason to believe that this region of the brain has been damaged in the overweight and that appetite can no longer serve as a self-control mechanism. It has been demonstrated that the region responsible for sending signals of hunger and satiety continues to function correctly in those with excess body fat. We don't eat in a balanced manner simply because we ignore the signals being sent by our central nervous system. Instead, we follow habits based on myths and erroneous beliefs, such as: eat very little even when you're still hungry; if possible, skip meals; feel guilty when hunger appears; reduce sugar consumption; eliminate fats from your diet, etc.

Only when you *unlearn* your current eating habits and *relearn* to listen to your body will you be cured of excess body fat.

This is obviously difficult and will not be achieved in a day, a week, or a month. But, after applying recommendations from this book, you will have the option of eating what your body asks for and reducing the excess fat.

16. Eating Without Discomfort

I hope I have convinced you that you must eat in order to permanently reduce excess body fat. Now I only need to mention a small detail that will save you pain, worry, and frustration.

What happens when someone on a diet starts eating normally again?

THE RE-FEEDING PHENOMENOM

At the end of World War Two, it was discovered in an unfortunate and accidental way what happens when a fasting individual begins eating all kinds of food. Some prisoners who had survived years of mistreatment in concentration camps, died tragically because of the care of their saviors. Their deaths were caused by severe digestive alterations when they were allowed to eat freely.

This reaction, known as the re-feeding phenomenon, was also observed in the overweight and described by Dr. Wayne Callaway. He reported that when an overweight person on a diet begins to eat food freely again, he unleashes reactions similar to those in famished prisoners in concentration camps. These include swelling of the abdomen, intense diarrhea, morning sickness with vomiting, and the formation of gases in the alimentary canal. Less dangerous, but more frightening to the overweight person, is a weight increase of up to 12 pounds in less than a week.

Many overweight people live in a self-appointed nutritional concentration camp.

Unfortunately, my new reduction strategy, the Bolio System described in section three, in which body fat is eliminated by eating all kinds of food, almost always produces the re-feeding phenomenon. This reaction can be reduced in such a way that in just a few days you will be eating all you want without causing gastrointestinal symptoms. For that purpose, I have devised a Recovery Phase, which is described in the first two weeks of the Bolio System.

The following are general recommendations to help you avoid the re-feeding phenomenon:

1. BEGIN WITH SMALL FOOD PORTIONS.

Those who have avoided beans will get diarrhea if they suddenly begin eating them in abundance. To reduce this possibility, start with very small portions. Gradually increase the quantities, and you will notice that in a few days you can eat all you want without any problem. If you have not enjoyed many food groups in a while, have patience, and soon you will be able to eat what you want without unwelcome side effects.

Those who experience digestive alterations such as colitis or gastritis will greatly reduce their symptoms by starting the Bolio System with weeks one and two (the Recovery Phase). By the third week, they will be able to enjoy almost all types of food without digestive symptoms.

2. EAT AS MANY TIMES A DAY AS POSSIBLE.

If you eat several times a day, continue with this excellent habit. Any type of food can be easily digested when taken in small and frequent portions. Eating one cracker a day for a year is of little concern, but eating 365 crackers in one shot will provoke unwelcome symptoms in anyone. If you have the bad habit of not eating between meals, learn to eat more frequently.

3. DO NOT PAY ATTENTION TO SELF-APPOINTED EXPERTS.

Although the recommendation to eat all kinds of food in order to lose excess body fat seems at first absurd, with time you will be convinced that this is the best option. Eating without restraint almost always produces guilt and fear in those with excess body fat. If you also pay attention to well-intentioned (but ill-informed) friends who consider themselves experts in this subject, you will not eat as indicated, you will not lose weight, and your friends will conclude that they were right.

Even if these self-proclaimed experts swear to you that carbohydrates make you fat, pay no attention to their comments and eat exactly what is indicated in the menu.

Excess body fat is one of the most complex diseases, and thousands of pages have been written about this subject. Fortunately for those with excess weight, the solution is really not complex. All you have to do is to learn to eat in a new manner.

4. DO NOT ANNOUNCE THE FACT THAT YOU ARE STARTING A WEIGHT-LOSS PLAN.

If you want to be completely briefed on all of the new strategies, fashionable doctors, teas, shakes, pills, and biorhythms, make public your commitment to reduce excess fat. You will surely hear on more than one occasion, "Don't waste your time! That plan is really useless! Look at how fat I am from eating everything I wanted! You would do a lot better with these marvelous products that I can sell you…"

Until you've seen the changes in your body (which become evident in approximately four weeks), do not try to convince others to follow this program. The result might well be that you are convinced to leave it. Later on, when your friends see that you have eliminated excess fat through eating, you will have a powerful weapon to convince them to read this book, so they can also learn to eat and be thin. (Do not lend them your book. Tell them to buy their own copy.)

5. TRY TO EAT WITHOUT FEELING GUILTY.

Some people find it almost impossible to eat freely without feeling guilt, fear, or even intense anguish.

Normally, human beings who eat apple pies will pass their food through their esophagus, stomach, small intestine, and colon. But those of us who have been on diet know for sure that there is a direct connection between our mouth and our waistline. Within five minutes of eating a piece of apple pie, we can feel the fat starting to accumulate around our belly.

I frequently joke with my patients about this feeling and call it "guilt fat", since patients feel they are definitely getting fatter even though they are losing weight and inches. Most people are surprised to learn that even though they *feel* fatter, their clothes fit better. When following the Bolio System, no one feels that he or she is losing excess fat. The changes can only be established through objective tests such as the measuring tape, the scale, and the way clothes fit.

The truth is that eating all kinds of food in a rational way will seldom cause your body to increase in either weight or inches.

If you find it impossible to eliminate an intense sensation of anguish every time you eat something that tastes good, keep in mind that the only way to be sure that eating will make you thin is by doing it. The day will come when you can sit down at the table to enjoy your food and become slender –and all without feeling guilty.

The Bolio System is divided into weeks. During the first weeks, the amount of food recommended will be moderated to reduce the re-feeding phenomenon. If you are currently on a strict weight-loss diet or are disciplined in applying even the strictest diets, you should follow recommendations for weeks one and two (the Recovery Phase). If you are not currently on a diet, you can start with weeks three, four, five, or six. As the program advances, you will increase the quantity and variety of the food you eat until you feel full and satisfied. You will be able to eat beans, pasta, whole wheat bread, non-diet soft drinks, bananas, avocadoes, almonds, peanuts, vegetable oils, cereals, pastry, pizzas and hamburgers. Sounds attractive, right?

Although a previous knowledge of the fundamental principles of the Bolio System is not necessary for the technique to work, understanding why it works will help you begin your program without inappropriate feelings of anxiety and guilt.

If you are like the majority of people who are trying to avoid gaining excess weight, you look on many foods with fear or even panic. Therefore, I recommend that you carefully re-read the first two sections of this book, so that you will be able to eat freely without fear or guilt.

The Bolio System recommendations outlined in part three are designed for those who can prepare their food at home. Those who frequently eat at restaurants will find more accessible techniques in my book, *What the Naturally Skinny Do to Stay Skinny.*

17. Preparing To Change the Way You Eat

Changing habits is not an easy task, but neither is it impossible to achieve. To successfully eliminate excess fat, your objectives need to be clearly established.

First, you must wholeheartedly embrace the idea that there is no "after the program." It is indispensable that you bury forever behaviors that lead to the accumulation of excess body fat, substituting them for eating habits that contribute to a slender body. The following is a list of habits that every "formerly overweight" person should have in his or her life:

1. Eat something when you wake up.
2. Always eat breakfast.
3. Eat something in mid-morning.
4. Always eat lunch.
5. Eat something in mid-afternoon.
6. Always eat dinner.
7. Eat something before going to sleep.
8. Include all nutrients in your menu.
9. Moderate the consumption of animal fat.
10. Use vegetable oils with prudence.

The most important tool to achieve permanent fat loss is patience. If you are desperately seeking to lose weight quickly, you are denying yourself the opportunity to modify your eating patterns and permanently lose weight.

Do not be discouraged by the slow rate of weight loss on the Bolio System. Sooner or later you will obtain the desired result. Impatience will only send you back to "miracle plans" that will eventually cause greater fat accumulation.

If you feel it is absolutely essential to obtain a spectacular figure in 24 hours and not obtaining it will cause you great frustration, you are in more need of psychological support than a weight-loss program.

Note also that a slender body will not give you immediate happiness. That is more easily obtained through chocolate ice cream. (Remember that fats liberate endorphins and endorphins give you sexual-like pleasure.)

The nutritional recommendations in this book will seem at first rather insipid. You must learn to enjoy many new foods and ways of preparing food, and before this is achieved, the menu will seem somewhat boring. A diet rich in saturated fat is naturally tastier. Therefore, you must be prepared to tolerate frustration. If you do not immediately become as thin as you want to be in spite of being disciplined in following this boring program, it does not matter. The day will come when you will surely be thin. And, with time, this insipid diet will become very pleasant to your taste.

If you recognize that you have a low tolerance for frustration, it would be better, before trying to modify your eating habits, that you seek professional help from a psychologist or through self-help groups such as Overeaters Anonymous. Overeaters Anonymous very wisely does not promote any particular diet, but rather addresses physical, emotional, and spiritual well-being. Its website is www.oa.org.

There are other matters that you must take into account when increasing the number of occasions that you eat:

The first one is that you will be adding more work to your already burdened life style. Since this is a program which must preferably be prepared at home and carried along during the day, you must take into account these situations. I always explain to my patients that it is much easier to lose weight by not eating than by eating. When you lose weight by eating you must: go to the supermarket, choose the right foods, stand in line to pay, carry your food home, store it, wash your hands, prepare it, cook it, wash your hands, measure it, eat it, dispend it, wash your hands and teeth, wash the dishes, pick up the kitchen, etc. When you don't eat all you have to do is just that.

Second, you must take into account that you need to take extra care of oral hygiene. Instead of washing your mouth three times a day, you will probably have to hike it up at least to five times per day. Check with your dentist that you are indeed washing your teeth correctly.

A welcome benefit that you will find is spending less money on food. It has been calculated that people throw away somewhere between 20 and 30% of the food that they buy, and this will not happen since your portions will be precisely measured.

Taken all this into account, losing weight by eating is definitely more rewarding in a social, emotional, and biological standpoint. It is really quite worth the effort. So don't despair, and continue with this program even when it does increase your daily work load.

PART THREE
THE BOLIO SYSTEM

Week One
(RECOVERY PHASE)

The recommendations prescribed in the first two weeks are for those who are currently on a strict weight-loss program and wish to switch to the Bolio System. You can also apply these recommendations if you are very disciplined and strict with any diet. If you are not at this moment on a diet, or if you are not disciplined or do not want to be disciplined at this moment, then start with recommendations prescribed for week three and begin following the plan from there. If you start the Recovery Phase and find it difficult to apply and/or feel very hungry, immediately advance to week three.

The recommendations for these first two weeks are intended to provide a phase-in period for people who are already on a strict diet. They are designed to reduce the unwelcome symptoms of the re-feeding phenomenon (swelling, diarrhea, gas, etc.; see chapter fifteen), to minimize intestinal problems, to minimize the possibility of weight gain, and to begin reducing excess body fat. I have observed fantastic results in people who have switched from a low-carbohydrate diet to this technique, for instance.

You can also apply this program if you wish to observe very quick changes in weight and measurements. However, these two weeks are much stricter than the rest of the program.

The basic structure of the Recovery Phase is a low fat, high complex carbohydrate plan. According to recent studies, programs with this structure will not reduce high triglyceride blood levels. How can you know if you have this problem?

Only through laboratory testing can you be sure that your triglycerides are normal. I will insist again that you have a physical check-up with your doctor before starting this, or any other program that modifies your eating pattern, even when you feel healthy.

If you have high triglycerides in the blood, it does not mean that you cannot apply the Recovery Phase, but you must be carefully monitored by your doctor. I have even given this plan to diabetics with fantastic results, but then again, this was done under strict surveillance.

Why would this high carbohydrate program work on elevated triglycerides and/or blood glucose? The main difference of this plan from other programs is that you are prompted to eat every two to three hours, and that pattern in itself tends to reduce triglycerides, blood glucose *and* cholesterol.

Never change your eating pattern if you have diabetes, hypertension or any other disease unless you have the permission of your doctor and his strict surveillance.

THE YOGURT SHAKE

The foundational food for the first two weeks is a shake. To prepare it with yogurt you need the following formula:

Women	
plain non-fat yogurt (0% fat)	4 fl oz
honey	4 tsp
olive oil	1 tsp
almonds, roasted	4 each

Men	
plain non-fat yogurt (0% fat)	6 fl oz
honey	4 tsp
olive oil	1 tsp
almonds, roasted	6 each

You must add honey, olive oil, and nuts to your yogurt to avoid weight regain. I recommend that you use Italian olive oil, since it tastes better when combined with yogurt.

If you have intolerance for milk products, try lactose-free yogurt or any of the following options:

PROTEIN POWDER SHAKES

An extraordinary shake can be obtained with soy protein isolate, which, in my experience, leads to greater reductions in fat than any other beverage. Soy protein isolate can be obtained in most health food stores. You can balance this product using the following formula:

Soy protein isolate (powder)	2 tsp (10 grams)
almonds, roasted	8 each
honey	4 tsp
Water	as needed

Instead of soy protein you can use milk based protein. This is the formula:

100% whey protein (powder)	2 tsp (10 grams)
Banana, medium	1 each
Sunflower oil	1 tsp
Water	as needed

You can also prepare the following shake with egg whites (egg protein):

egg whites	2 ounces
olive oil	1 tsp.
Banana, medium	1 each
Cook the egg whites with olive oil and eat your banana on the side.	

These formulas are identical for men and women, with the difference that men will probably take more shakes.

These are only a few examples. There are many protein supplements on the market and any one of these can be used in the Bolio System, but you need to add certain elements to make them work properly with this plan. If you have a special protein supplement that you wish to use with this program, contact me through the Internet, and I will calculate what ingredients must be added to make it work. The website address is: www.drbolio.com or www.esbelto.com (Spanish version).

As a general rule, protein based shakes result in greater fat mobilization (burn more fat, turn more fat into energy) than yogurt; as long as you prepare the formula with precision.

COMMERCIALY PREPARED BALANCED DRINKS

You can replace previously marked shakes with any beverage that is balanced.

How can you tell if a beverage has the proper balance of macro nutrients?

First, identify the total grams protein under "Nutrition Facts" or "Nutrition Information" on the label. If you multiply this amount by 0.9, it will give you the number of grams of fat that the beverage should contain to have the proper balance. Now multiply the number of grams of protein by 4 to get the grams of carbohydrates the beverage should contain.

For example, Ensure Plus® contains 13 grams of protein. When you multiply 13 by 0.9, you get 11.7, which is the amount of fat needed to balance this protein. Since the beverage contains 11 grams of fat, it is close enough to be considered balanced. When you now multiply 13 by 4, you get 52, which is the amount of carbohydrates that this drink should have. Since the beverage contains 50 grams of carbohydrates, it is a balanced drink.

This formula can be applied to any beverage found on the market. Some other drinks that are balanced or close to balanced according to the formula are chocolate-flavored Silk® soy milk and Walgreen's® nutritional drink.

Any beverage that is not balanced, according to the formula, is inappropriate for this program.

DAILY PORTIONS

The yogurt shake must be taken four times a day. If you're still hungry after four servings (and you probably will be), add as many alternative protein shakes (soy protein, whey protein, etc.) and commercially prepared balanced drinks (chocolate flavored Silk® soy milk, Ensure Plus®, etc.) as you need until your hunger is satisfied. Reducing intake in the hope that this will accelerate weight loss may only lead to malnutrition, which sooner or later will reduce your body's ability to convert fat into energy, thus regaining any weight and inches that you lost.

How much is too much? I do not recommend more than four yogurt shakes per day. Protein shakes and balanced drinks such as soy protein isolate can be taken freely, in whatever quantities you wish. In fact, it was through the use of these products that I discovered how eating in abundance can make you thin.

Take your first shake as soon as you wake up, before having a bath or shower or getting dressed. If you are in the habit of staying in bed for a few minutes after you wake up, leave the shake next to your bed before you go to sleep. If taking time for a shake is going to make you late for work, wake up earlier.

Drink your last shake immediately before going to sleep. Many people read a book or watch television in bed before going to sleep. In that case, have your last shake only when you are ready to go to sleep.

Program your shakes at regular intervals throughout the day (with no more than six hours between servings). Most people have a shake every three to four hours. If you sleep more than six hours a day, be especially careful to have your first serving immediately after waking up and your last serving just before going to sleep.

Some people find the four yogurt shakes excessive. If this is the case, you can cut the portion in half and take eight half shakes instead of four: the more occasions you eat, the faster you will lose fat.

Several options are available to you if you are going to be away from home during the day. In order to keep your shake cool, you can mix the ingredients using cold yogurt, or you can add ice to the blender. A thermos can also help to keep the temperature low enough to prevent fermentation. If you decide to use powdered protein supplements, you can prepare your shake the same way you would at home with water, a spoon, and a little patience.

The shakes are the foundational food for the first two weeks, but new food groups will be added to the menu each day to go along with the shakes.

FIRST DAY

Plain non-fat yogurt with honey, olive oil, and roasted almonds (that is, a shake)

This is, for many, the hardest day of all. Aside from the yogurt, alternatives and commercial balanced drinks, only water is permitted. Be sure to drink a minimum of eight glasses of water per day.

If you find this day overly difficult, skip to the recommendations for the second, third, or fourth day and start the program from there.

Twenty-four hours of relative fasting is no big deal. Most dieters have already tried more drastic programs. Besides, the shakes will help to reduce your food cravings, although it is impossible to stop missing all of those tasty and fatty foods we are all so used to. It is difficult to stop eating addictive foods, but it is not impossible. And there is no need to feel hungry since you can have as many shakes as you want. Remember to also drink at least eight glasses of water this day.

SECOND DAY

Add melon, papaya, watermelon, and/or pineapple, mixed with equal parts of water.

Aside from the shakes, you must prepare a second mix consisting of equal parts of water and one or more of the fruits mentioned above. In other words, if you want four ounces of melon, blend it with four ounces of water. You may drink as much as you want as often as you want whenever you want. It is best to drink this several times a day, and the total daily amount should add up to no less than eight glasses. The more you drink, the easier it will be to continue avoiding other foods.

If you are a woman who has experience with miracle pills, diets and massages, you know that it is almost impossible to selectively reduce fat from the buttocks and hips. Fat disappears from the abdomen, breasts, and legs, but there seems to be no solution for those prominent hips and thick thighs. However, there is a way to eliminate fat from this region; drink this fruit-and-water mixture (preferably using papaya) every hour, drinking as much as you want. This will lead to a preferential reduction of fat from the hips and buttocks. To date, this is the fastest way that I know to selectively reduce this region.

Waist measurement will be reduced by following recommendations for week three and following. Reduction of the waist measurement (elimination of fat from this area) is also encouraged by the consumption of green leafy vegetables.

THIRD DAY

Add all kinds of cooked vegetables, on at least three occasions throughout the day.

You can include potatoes, corn, carrots, beets, and any other tuberous vegetables. These are foods that low carb advocates link to excess body fat, but don't be afraid to eat as much as you want of them. How much is too much? There is no limit. Remember that your food intake has been very restricted during the previous 48 hours, and you have earned the right to eat until you feel full.

Limiting the quantities of these vegetables because of fear will only make you lose very little body fat. Do not try to "improve on" this program by eating only small quantities. If you are going to make your own rules, you might as well be on any other fat-loss program. These first days of relative fasting are intended to reduce the re-feeding phenomenon, not to generate quick weight loss.

If you have preferential accumulation of fat around the waist, then use as much green leaf vegetables (lettuce, spinach, celery, etc.) as you can at least three times a day and you will see how in less than one week, your fat starts to melt away.

Be creative and season your vegetables with salt, pepper, garlic, spices, or any another non-fat seasoning. You can even cook with chicken broth, as long as you separate the fat from the broth. Once the fat has been eliminated, you can use any type of broth to cook your vegetables. Any restricted-eating program is more tolerable if food is prepared with the right spices. You must learn to intensely enjoy vegetables, and this can be achieved with seasonings that do not contain fat. Keep in mind that it is always easier to complete a pleasant task than an unpleasant one.

Of course, you should continue to take as many shakes as you need to feel satisfied (at least four a day), as well as at least eight glasses of the fruit-and-water mixture.

FOURTH DAY

Add all kinds of raw vegetables, on at least two occasions.

Although we enjoy eating vegetables, we aren't always in the habit of eating them raw. It's worthwhile for you to learn to savor the pleasure of eating a well-prepared salad. Have a salad at least twice a day.

Although I do not know the scientific reason behind the following recommendation, I can assure you that it works: The more green leaf vegetables that are eaten, the more inches you will lose from your waistline. If you're in a hurry to lose fat around the waist, eat green vegetables at least three times a day (including breakfast, as they do in the kibbutzim in Israel).

The only vegetable you should not include in your salads is avocado. In the strict sense, it is a fruit, although many add it to salty dishes. Avocado has a high fat content; therefore, you need to ration how much you eat of it. It will be added in the second week of the program.

Remember to continue to have your shakes, fruit-and-water mix, and cooked vegetables.

FIFTH DAY

Add melon, papaya, watermelon, and/or pineapple, on at least four occasions.

These are sometimes called "diet" fruits, since they contain a great volume of water and a minimum of calories. By this day, you can generally eat as much of these fruits as you wish without having to mix them with water and without triggering the re-feeding phenomenon.

On this fifth day, you must continue to include all previously recommended foods; the cooked and raw vegetables and at least four shakes.

Don't make the mistake of eating only what is to be added each day (for example, only salads on day four, or only fresh fruit on day five) since this may increase malnutrition and limit the conversion of body fat. (If you try this, you will lose more weight, but fewer inches.)

Women who are using the hip-reduction program can eat papaya every hour without having to mix it with water.

SIXTH DAY

Add all types of fruit, on at least four occasions.

You are now ready to add a significant quantity of calories to your diet. Do you wish to eat bananas? Go ahead. Or are mangoes the most addictive fruit that you can think of? Have as many as you desire. You deserve it, for you have significantly restricted your food options for five days.

On this sixth day, you will add elements to your diet that are prohibited or severely limited in almost any other fat-loss program. Don't worry. By now the scale and measuring tape will have already demonstrated the excellent results you are receiving from this program, and they will continue to do so as long as you eat without fear.

Eat any type of fruit on at least four occasions on this day. Eating fruit less frequently will only result in a slower rate of excess fat loss. More importantly, remember that it is frequent eating that leads to the loss of excess body fat. Diets that recommend only three meals a day (especially if they are very low in calories) may lead to loss of muscle and normal fat. If you are a woman looking for a better figure, it makes no sense to apply a program that will result in a flabby body and sagging breasts.

If you eat fruits more than four times a day, you will notice an even greater loss of excess body fat. But if four times a day seems difficult, try very hard to maintain at least that level.

Eating frequently has such impressive effects on the metabolism that results are observed with almost any type of food group. I have even seen how eating apple pie every hour results in loss of body fat.

SEVENTH DAY

Add all kinds of pasta, on at least two occasions.

This is the last day of the week. We will end this week by adding another food group that has been greatly criticized and yet holds extraordinary potential for reducing body fat–pasta. Doesn't that sound wonderful, to lose inches off your waist by eating a large plate of spaghetti?

Although pasta is a processed food, the body digests it as if it were a pear (a fruit with a very low glycemic index) and as if it contained high quantities of fiber. All of these properties make pasta an excellent reducing element **as long as you don't add fat when cooking it.**

You can buy pre-cooked pasta which is very easy to prepare. You can also toast your pasta in a Teflon pan, and then cook it the usual way. Another possibility is to add pasta to boiling water. You can smother it in tomato juice, as well as any other seasoning.

On this day, of course, you are still taking at least four shakes, all types of fruit, plus prescribed servings of cooked and raw vegetables.

During this first week, most people experience a significant loss of weight and inches. Some lose up to two inches around the hips. Almost everyone who participates in this program is fascinated by results, especially by seeing how food that is supposedly fattening causes fat loss.

However, pay no attention to the weight loss you have achieved this week. The recommendations for this week are intended to help you to eat all kinds of food without experiencing unpleasant symptoms such as stomach upset. They will not help you to permanently eliminate excess body fat. Permanent fat loss is obtained only through permanent changes to your eating habits, not by any single diet plan.

If you followed the program and gained weight during this week, this means that you are severely malnourished. You should immediately seek the help of a doctor and/or nutritionist, who will guide you through the re-feeding phenomenon. You can also ask for support at: www.drbolio.com or www.esbelto.com (Spanish version).

A word of caution, do not repeat any day even when for any reason you did not follow it perfectly and/or you added something that was not programmed. You must continue to add food groups according to the traced progressive plan.

Said another way, by the end of the week *you must have finished with all recommendations*, even if for any reason you were not very strict in its application.

I know of a patient who was so motivated by the changes of her friends that she stubbornly continued to repeat days one and two since, for some reason or another, there was always something extra added to the plan. The only thing she obtained was under nutrition and greater fat accumulation.

These programs are not a test of will power.

If the Recovery Phase does not fit you, leave it and apply recommendations of week three to nine. If even these recommendations seem difficult to follow, try the plan outlined in my other book *What the Naturally Skinny Do to Stay Skinny*.

If you cannot follow *any* program, don't worry. I have found that even despite the desperate attitude of those who come to my office to lose weight, it turns out that sooner or later everyone discovers that there is more to life than just dieting.

Therefore your best option is to temporarily forget about even trying to start a program.

What you can and should do is increase the number of occasions that you eat and add or increase any of the wise choices listed on chapter 14 to your daily plan.

Week Two
(RECOVERY PHASE continued)

The menu prescribed for the first week will cover your body's minimum daily needs, but it lacks an element important to anyone's program: variety.

In this second week, we will add other types of food to previous recommendations. This may slow down the loss of inches and weight. Don't let this worry you. Speed of fat loss is the least important factor in a sensible weight-control program. **Your main goal is permanent fat loss and not a quick and transitory weight change.**

Always keep in mind that anyone can start a severely restricted weight-loss program, but very few finish it. That is why it is necessary to apply a plan that offers sufficient and pleasant food over a more limited program that generates greater fat loss. Choose the program that you can stick to in the long run in order to obtain permanent loss of inches and weight.

Let me phrase it another way. I have never yet been able to create a program where I can say: "This is what is best for you, but don't follow any recommendation since you will lose excess fat anyway." The best method in the world is absolutely useless when not applied. Continuing to use a very restricted eating pattern that favors quick weight loss will keep you from enjoying a liberal program that teaches you to eat in a healthy and prudent way. When are you going to learn to eat to be thin if you spend the rest of your life limiting yourself in order to lose weight quickly or for fear of gaining it back?

The first week is structured in such a way that you are always eating more complex carbohydrates than fats. When you take four women's yogurt shakes, two cups of cooked pasta, three cups of vegetables (including potatoes, beets, carrots, etc.), four cups of melon, one banana, one apple, one pear, and one orange, you are eating almost 2,000 calories per day, but only 17% of those calories are coming from fat. This macronutrient distribution is very similar to Chinese eating patterns where obesity is rare.

Diets with this structure will definitely produce spectacular and satisfactory weight changes, but in the long run they can cause metabolic instability (i.e., starvation mode). People are very happy with these diets, but doctors are not. In order to generate a metabolically stable rate of fat loss, you need to have at least 25% of calories in your diet come from fat (and preferably between 27% and 33%). The danger of continuing with very low fat diets is that even though you will certainly make you lose more weight and inches in the short run, in the long run you may regain all the excess fat that you have lost.

That is why we must add fats to our diet in this second week.

Many may feel fear when adding these food groups to their menu. This is natural, and it is not surprising, but don't let fear keep you from following this program and achieving the weight loss you want.

By now, your body should be ready to digest more fats without suffering any unpleasant side effects. If these do appear, there is a possibility that you have a concurrent intestinal disease. If you notice abdominal pain, diarrhea, constipation, or gas, you should make an appointment with your doctor, who will carefully check you and prescribe an adequate treatment. The gradual addition of fiber and fat to your diet should not cause intestinal symptoms.

There is also a possibility that you have irritable bowel syndrome. This problem is associated with a lack of physical activity and/or an inappropriate diet (high in fat and low in fiber), but is most closely associated with chronic stress. If you are under great and chronic stress, you must learn new ways to manage it. There will be no effective treatment of irritable bowel syndrome as long as you let stress run free in your life.

If the unpleasant symptoms are minor, continue with the program. With time, your stomach will adapt to this diet, and the symptoms will generally disappear in one or two weeks.

FIRST DAY

Add boiled rice on at least two occasions.

From a metabolic viewpoint, pasta burns more body fat than rice does since it has a lower glycemic index. But for many people rice is more appealing. Variety will also make this program easier to follow.

Remember that rice must be prepared without adding oil. Perhaps flavor will be different, but you also have the option of preparing it with good seasoning. Eat either rice or pasta on at least two occasions this day. Alternatively, you can eat rice **and** pasta, on two occasions each, for a total of four occasions. If you eat more frequently, you will notice a greater loss of inches.

Remember that, besides the rice and/or pasta, you must continue to eat salads, cooked vegetables, all kinds of fruits, and at least four shakes.

Learn to determine your body's needs. If you have lived with food restrictions for years, it is time to let your body speak. Be very attentive to any feeling of being full or satisfied, or you will run the risk of eating excessive quantities of a single food group, and not enough of the other groups.

Watch the quantities carefully. If necessary, serve the different food groups on separate small plates. You can use dessert plates instead of your usual dinnerware. If, after eating small quantities, you are still hungry, go ahead and eat a little more. You can eat as many servings as you want.

If hunger returns after a few hours, don't worry. Eat some more. When you eat several times a day, you lose inches faster.

As a general rule, if you are hungry one hour after eating something, you have taken too little. If more than three hours pass and you are still not hungry, then you have eaten too much.

Those who decide to eat very little, or on few occasions during the day, lose more weight but less body fat, and they lose it in places where they don't want to.

Remember that body fat is an indispensable element and that it is used in specific parts of our body, such as breasts in women and subcutaneous facial fat which gives you a youthful look. If you change this plan and eat less than recommended, breasts could shrink and sag and you could end up looking very, very old by the end of the program.

This program has nothing to do with quantities (calories). That is why you must listen to your body and let your Center of Appetite and Satiety dictate when you have eaten enough and when you should eat a little more.

Eating as much as you want to lose weight and inches is a marvelous experience that should be savored by all those who have at some time in their life limited their food intake for fear of growing fat.

SECOND DAY:

Add one ration of vegetable fat.

The human body is built from fat. A third part of each cell's membrane wall is made up of fat, and 80% of the brain is composed of fat molecules. Women's mammary glands as well as hips obtain their consistency and shape from fat. If a woman has less than 12% of fat in her body, she will stop menstruating and become sterile. Fat is indispensable in the human body.

Many people may feel fear when adding fats to their menu, especially after being informed that they are part of the problem of excess body fat. Yet you must eat enough quantities of this food group, or you will run the risk of gaining back all the inches and weight you have lost, and even more. A very low fat diet will also damage the skin and the immune system.

Choose one of the following:

Vegetable Fat Rations	
A vegetable fat ration is equal to:	
Vegetable oil (for salads)	1 tsp.
Olive oil (for cooking and/or salads)	1 tsp.
Cocoa, dry powder, unsweetened	1 ounce (28 grams)
Peanut butter	1 tsp.
Almonds, roasted	8 each
Cashews	8 each
Pistachios	12 each
Raw peanuts	12 each
Avocado	¼ medium size
Canned olives	1.6 ounces (50 grams)
Mayonnaise	1 tsp. (5 grams)

THIRD DAY

Add a second vegetable fat ration, for a total of two rations in 24 hours.

Although you can eat these two small rations of fat on one occasion, you will lose excess fat quicker if you have them on two occasions. This will also help you to control your triglyceride and cholesterol levels.

Remember that olive oil is the best oil to use in cooking. To calculate the quantity of fat that is absorbed when cooking, take into account that fried rice or pasta will absorb one tsp. of oil for every half cup. This means that if you eat one cup of fried rice, you have already eaten your two rations of fat.

FOURTH DAY

Add one ration of animal fat.

It is necessary that human beings eat certain quantities of animal fat.

Without saturated fats, a series of hormones indispensable for our survival would not exist. Brain cells are built using animal fat. Sexual hormones, as well as cortisone, are also created from saturated fats.

Even for a body with a great reservoir of these elements, the long-term effect of completely eliminating saturated fats from diet is not known. Therefore, it is most prudent to continue taking them. This is why small quantities of animal fat have been added to the Bolio System quite quickly, in just the second week.

Animal Fat Rations	
An animal fat ration is equal to:	
Butter	1 tsp.
Lard	1 tsp.
Cream	1 tbsp.
Bacon	1 small strip

These elements make food more enjoyable since it becomes tastier when we add them to our menu. This is a natural tendency. Therefore, take care not to exceed the prescribed rations of saturated fat.

How do strawberries with cream sound? Or do vegetables sautéed in butter appeal to you?

If you find it impossible to control quantities, stop taking them temporarily and add them back into your menu from the fifth week on.

FIFTH DAY

Add a second animal fat ration, for a total of two rations in 24 hours.

Even though you can take these two rations on one occasion, it is wise to distribute them over two occasions. If animal fats tempt you to add excessive amounts, use your will power to eat only what is recommended.

SIXTH AND SEVENTH DAY

Make no changes.

You have two days to play with your newly added animal and vegetable fat rations. You can eat them raw (for example, sour cream over cooked spinach) or use them to cook a special dish.

Use your imagination to make this program as pleasant as possible. Prepare your rice with olive oil, and save your animal fat rations so you can season your vegetables with bacon or butter.

Two rations of each fat group may not seem enough for those who are accustomed to a high-fat diet. But taking into account the fat from four women's yogurt shakes and the four extra portions, you are taking at least 55 grams of total fat per day. From a metabolic point of view, that constitutes the minimum daily requirement of human beings.

How about adding chocolate to your yoghurt, or simply mixing it with water?

In your daily diet, continue to include cooked and raw vegetables, pasta and/or rice, all types of fruit, and a minimum of four shakes.

Congratulations! By now you are eating a variety of foods high in complex carbohydrates and small portions of animal and vegetable fat. The idea that these food groups make you fat by now should be buried in the past.

Some will observe spectacular reductions in weight and inches. I have seen people lose more than three inches off their measurements during these first two weeks of the Bolio System. This response, however, is uncommon. The majority will obtain a slow but satisfactory loss of two to three pounds of body fat, or about one inch off their measurements.

I know of a lady that was so happy with her program that she decided to stay on Week Two as a permanent eating style. She lost all her excess weight, which was over 80 pounds, in a permanent and healthy way.

I do not recommend that you do this, for it is my philosophy that you obtain and maintain a stable and healthy weight with a program that includes **all food groups in your daily meal plan.**

Others may obtain minimum or null changes. This happens in about 10% to 12% of cases. If this is your situation, take into account that, even if your figure has not been modified, you have had the opportunity of eating an abundance of food groups that you had considered prohibited or sinful in the past.

Why do weight and measurements remain stable in some people? This depends on the degree of malnutrition present when you start this program. The Starvation Mode appears in obese individuals precisely because for a long time they have applied deficient diets in spite of being surrounded by an abundance of good food. Because of these long-term deficient diets, their bodies' survival mechanisms have been activated, making it impossible for them to lose weight in spite of severely restricting their food intake.

If these two weeks made you gain weight (this happens in 4% to 6% of cases), it means that you have severe malnutrition that must be treated by a doctor and/or a dietitian. This professional will recommend a special program that will help you get through the re-feeding phenomenon and may even prescribe some medication such as a diuretic.

Week Three

Those who follow recommendations of weeks one and two can lose anywhere between two to six pounds of body fat and one to three inches off their measurements. Some will lose more, others nothing at all. This is inevitable since each person loses fat at a different rate.

If you followed recommendations of weeks one and two and noticed minimal changes, be firm and continue with recommendations of the remaining weeks of the Bolio System. This program is definitely not the fastest in regards to short-term weight loss, but it will help you lose excess fat in a healthy and permanent manner.

Recommendations for weeks one and two have no resemblance to people's usual daily eating habits. This is why we must change the structure of the plan in week three. Any successful long-term program should propose recommendations that come as close as possible to people's usual eating habits. This way adherence is improved, as well as long-term results.

Each country or region has its own particular pattern of scheduling meals throughout the day. Latin countries usually have their heaviest meal between 1:00 and 3:00 p.m., while in the United States and Europe the heaviest meal is eaten late in the afternoon.

Latin countries have many excellent traditions involving food. For years, people in these countries ate five meals a day. Unfortunately, this changed when they imported the American way of life and began eating only breakfast, lunch, and dinner.

I had a great advantage in that I began working on the problem of excess body fat in my native country, Mexico. In first place, Mexicans are used to eating more than three times a day. More significantly, they have minimal discipline in regard to eating habits. This forced me to be creative and develop a very flexible and easy-to-follow program to eliminate excess body fat. The result is the Bolio System, in which you can lose excess fat by eating all types of food.

You will find a major change of lifestyle during lunch, when most people usually eat a small portion of animal protein accompanied with some bread portion (sandwiches, hamburgers, pizzas, etc.) This has been changed for beans, chickpeas, etc. There are various reasons for making use of this option:

1. In my personal experience, people will loose excess body fat much faster with this high vegetable protein program (usually labeled the Mediterranean Diet) than with a high animal protein balanced diet.

2. These programs usually reduce total cholesterol, triglycerides, uric acid and hypertension much better than with high animal protein balanced diets.

3. People seem to feel much better with this program than with a balanced diet based on animal protein; there is a general sensation of wellness reported by most patients.

4. The preferential loss of abdominal fat will usually be much faster with this program than with a balanced high animal protein diet.

If you feel lunchtime is very strange, please apply the program for at least three weeks before changing to other options. If after three weeks you still prefer different meals at lunch, don't hesitate to contact us and we will gladly balance out any meal that you decide to use during the afternoon.

This is one great advantage of the Bolo System over many other programs, since you can use ANY MEAL THAT YOU DESIRE to lose excess body fat. In the Bolio System, there are no forbidden plates.

We can be reached at:

www.drbolio.com (English version)
www.esbelto.com (Spanish version)

THE "PERFECT" PROGRAM: A BALANCED DIET

If you want to set on fire an extremely torrid discussion, just try to get obesity experts to agree on the "perfect" diet for obesity management. Some will state that the best option is a high protein, low carbohydrate, high fat diet. Others will insist on a high carbohydrate, normal protein, and low fat diet. If you add all the possible options for a high, normal, or low macronutrient program, then you can sum up just how many opinions exist around dietary obesity treatment.

Fortunately, recommendations for the general healthy population are less diverse. According to international health organizations, we should receive approximately 55% of our daily energy requirements in the form of carbohydrates, 15% from protein, 10% or less from saturated fats, and 20% or more from vegetable fats. A proper diet should also include at least 25 grams of fiber every day.

In concordance with this criteria a diet will usually be labeled high in carbohydrates when it contains more than 60% of these macronutrients, a high protein diet more than 18% and a high fat diet, more than 35%.

Since the statement that eating makes you skinny is, to say it mildly, controversial, I decided to follow the nutritional recommendations for the general population. My line of thinking was that if an obese individual had to eat to be thin, then he should follow a program identical to those recommended for the general healthy population.

What did I find with this program?

That over 80% of obese and overweight individuals slowly reduced their excess fat. Even people with normal weight and measurements lost any unsightly fat that they had. In my experience, this is the prefect program that reduces those last 5 pounds of body fat that were so hard to lose.

Most important, that a preferential loss of abdominal body fat ensued **without losing tone or consistency of glutei in men and women and breast in women.**

Patients referred a sensation of satiety where most cravings disappeared. That is to say, there was no suffering with this program.

There was a reduction of blood glucose, uric acid, cholesterol and triglycerides. Blood pressure was also reduced, especially on people with hypertension.

Hair became thicker and silkier, fingernails became firmer, facial wrinkles were reduced (disciplined people will look ten to twenty years younger); fat in cheeks went down, as well as fat in lower mandible. Surprisingly, breasts in women as well as glutes in men and women became firmer (especially with the higher calorie programs).

To my knowledge, no other program in the world can generate abdominal fat loss while at the same time increasing consistency and shape of breasts (in women) and gluteus.

People referred more energy, a more peaceful state of mind, less stress, better sleep and better mental concentration during the day.

Sexual drive as well as intensity was almost always increased as well as fertility. As a matter of fact, many women with primary fertility (that is to say, they had not gotten pregnant despite trying to do so) would become happy mothers.

Take this recommendation very seriously if you are not looking for a pregnancy: check with your doctor for the highest possible protection from pregnancy since fertility is highly increased.

I even had the opportunity of treating people who were cured of cancer and insulin dependent brittle diabetic women who stabilized their disease and gave birth to normal weight children (endocrinologists will say *wow* to this last statement).

I am not stating that this program is a miracle cure for every possible disease, since it is not. And I am not writing this to convince anyone to apply my system. You must not follow this program to cure yourself of anything, since this is a process that must be directed and overseen by a physician. When you do decide to follow these recommendations, it is because you have concluded that changing eating habits is your best option. But then, of course, it is fantastic to know that you can reap so many benefits by just applying a balanced program.

How can anyone without a doctorate in nutrition know if he or she is eating a properly balanced meal? Over five weeks of the Bolio System, I developed 35 different daily nutritional plans.

Every program fully complies with the criteria for a balanced meal cited above. This is why you will find some "strange" ingredients such as specific cereals, oil mixtures, and a lunch based on beans and chickpeas. This was made so that you receive at least 90% of the dietary reference intake (DRI) of vitamins and minerals. Those with special needs (such as women, who are pregnant, breast feeding or are in menopause) must consult their physician before starting this or any other program since different intake of macro and micronutrients are required.

I also recommend that you add two pearls of cod liver oil and 500mg of vitamin C twice a day.

If you carefully measure all ingredients, you will obtain a balanced meal plan that favors faster and more aesthetic results.

You will also find that the program is basically a one week plan that changes slightly from one week to another. The main differences between daily programs is that calories are gradually increased, starting with 1,200 on Monday of week three and ending with 2,200 on Sunday of week seven.

I want to emphasize that the Bolio System has nothing to do with calories.

This means that instead of starting in week three or four, you can start with recommendations of week seven, where maximum nutriments are recommended. The only risk with doing this is that if you are malnourished, the re-feeding phenomenon (with the resulting weight gain) might be triggered. This is not a great problem, but people are usually so afraid of the scale that they might decide to leave this program because of the weight gain in spite of the fact that they are losing inches off their measurements.

Also, I have observed in clinical practice that those who have been constantly on diets will usually not tolerate high-calorie diets at first. If they do attempt to have more than 2000 calories per day, they will not only feel that food is excessive, but may also develop intestinal symptoms such as swelling and cramps.

My recommendation is that women start with week three, and men with week four. If these recommendations keep you very hungry and you constantly have to add "hunger tamers" (see below), jump to one of the higher weeks until you find the program which keeps you satisfied, but not overfed.

Most people who start with weeks three or four will feel very satisfied for some time, but sooner or later will need more food. When this happens, they must advance to the next week. That is to say, if you feel fine with a specific week, repeat recommendations for that week as many times as you wish. When hunger strikes, you must advance to the following week, which includes more variety and abundance of food.

The presence of hunger and cravings are marvelous events which indicate that you are permanently ridding yourself of excess fat.

HUNGER TAMERS

Each person has his own personal food requirements that differ from everyone else's. Nutritional requirements even change from day to day in the same person. We will feel very hungry some days and on other days have only minimal appetite. This is a natural response that has been confirmed in various clinical studies. Unfortunately, this normal human trait may make recommendations for one day seem a real hardship, while on other days they may seem excessive.

In order to fill in these natural nutritional "fissures," you can add shakes indicated in week one (the Recovery Phase). Take as many as needed to eliminate hunger. With them, you can adapt the plan to your changing needs without upsetting the carefully designed balance of daily recommendations.

I will repeat the shake list:

Women	
plain non-fat yogurt (0% fat)	4 fl oz
Honey	4 tsp
olive oil	1 tsp
almonds, roasted	4 each

Men	
plain non-fat yogurt (0% fat)	6 fl oz
Honey	4 tsp
olive oil	1 tsp
almonds, roasted	6 each

Soy protein isolate	2 tsp (10 grams)
Banana, medium	1 each
Sunflower oil	1 tsp.
almonds, roasted	2 each
Honey	1 tsp
Water	as needed

100% whey protein	2 tsp (10 grams)
Banana, medium	1 each
Sunflower oil	1 tsp
Water	as needed

egg whites	2 ounces
olive oil	1 tsp.
Banana, medium	1 each
Cook the egg whites with olive oil and eat your banana on the side.	

Commercially prepared balanced drinks:

Chocolate flavored Silk® soy milk

Ensure® and Ensure Plus

Walgreens® nutritional drink

You can also freely add as much as you want of protein with low or no fat (non fat or 1% fat milk, plain non fat or 1% fat yogurt, non fat cheese, protein supplements, chicken or turkey breast without skin, fish, lean steak, etc.), all types of vegetables (potatoes, beets, carrots, etc.) and all types of fruit (bananas, mangos, etc.).

Just take into account that if you find yourself using many "hunger tamers", you must advance to the following week until you find the one where you require of these options once and at most, twice a day.

If you decide to add shakes, non fat protein, vegetables and/or fruit, you must still eat **all** recommended foods marked in each daily menu.

And if for some reason, you have a craving for a particular food, such as chocolate chip cookies, doughnuts, potato chips, etc., even after adding the "hunger tamers", go ahead and eat that craving, as long as you do it without fear or guilt. **But eating something that is not in the program is no excuse to reduce what is in the program, even if the extra snack left you without hunger.**

On certain occasions, people will feel the need to eat "something" but will be unable to precisely define their craving. In this case, drink a glass of water and wait for at least fifteen minutes before deciding what to snack. Dehydration seems to stunt our ability to perceive certain biologic needs such as cravings (yes, cravings have a *biological* as well as an *emotional* component).

In this regard, I recommend that you add at least four glasses of water to all daily program, just to be sure that you are well hydrated. In warm climates you may have to drink even more.

Some people will try to "compensate" cravings by subtracting fats and carbohydrates from their plan when they gorge on some dessert that was not programmed. This is forbidden in the Bolio System.

The Bolio System is based on the philosophy that you must always offer your body a balanced and healthy meal, no matter what disastrous decision you have previously made. Don't take so much of the craving that you are unable to eat recommended foods at the next meal.

MAXIMUM AND MINIMUM PORTIONS

Only one in 100 persons who follows this program will be able to eat all that is recommended in the seventh week. The majority find the portions of weeks five and six sufficient and even on occasion excessive.

When you find a week that keeps you satisfied, repeat it as many times as possible. For example, if week five is adequate, continue with it for at least five or six more weeks. Always keep in mind that protein, vegetables, fruits, and shakes are free and you can use them to fill up any extra need.

You can also repeat any day that you find easy and enjoyable to apply. Perhaps the menu recommended for Wednesday of week six is perfect for you. In this case, you would repeat Wednesday's recommendations **five times**, from Monday to Friday. Why only five times and not all week long? Because Saturday and Sunday should ideally be applied just as they are in order to learn to lose excess fat eating in restaurants.

Repeating recommendations of one day all week long can be much more practical than changing menus from one day to the other, but on the long run it is more boring and unfortunately you will also lose less abdominal fat than with variety.

How many times can you repeat the same week's or the same day's recommendations?

It has been reported that when a repetitive action is continued for at least three consecutive months, it usually becomes a habit. For example, those who avoid smoking for twelve weeks will usually quit the habit.

If you follow the Bolio System for nine weeks, fine. But if you extend it three to six more weeks, **it will yield even better long-term results**. By then you will be in the habit of eating healthy, satisfying meals, and able to continue that pattern indefinitely with no great difficulty.

The contrary can also be true, that is to say, you may find that at some point in the program, your appetite is drastically reduced. This is not very common, but it does happen: certain events such as depression, acute stress and/or an infectious disease may reduce your appetite.

If this happens, you can reduce your daily intake by going back to previous weeks. For example, if you are in Week Seven and suddenly feel that quantities are excessive, you should backtrack to a week that indicates less food (Weeks Two to Four).

A word of caution for those who feel the need to reduce their caloric intake: glutei and breasts (in women) **must stay in place and/or recuperate their firmness:**

It is extremely important that you obtain a **better looking body when applying this or any other fat loss program**. Low calorie diets will certainly make you lose weight and inches very quickly, but since they are not covering all your daily needs, they will also consume muscular mass, thus producing sagging muscles and skin. Believe me, bodies generated by very low calorie diets look really, really ugly when clothes are taken off.

HOW OBSESSIVE SHOULD I BE WHEN MEASURING MY PORTIONS?

In a study carried out with a restaurant that prepared menus with mathematical precision, the average loss of weight was four pounds per week. This was obtained with a 1,500 calorie diet and ad libitum (eat as much as you want) balanced shakes. This result is spectacular, especially since it was accompanied with a rapid loss of weight **and** inches.

Carefully measuring and weighing portions is certainly burdensome, but you get the added benefit of a much faster elimination of excess body fat.

Therefore, it is up to you to decide just how careful you should be with measurements. If being very strict generates stress, then work with approximate portions. But if being "picky" is enjoyable to you, then go ahead and do it.

In the Bolio System you can eat more than what is indicated but not less that what is marked. This means that you should be very obsessive in making sure that you are adding exactly what is indicated **plus** whatever your body craves. Said another way, cravings are and must be a natural part of your program. Food measurements are not meant to substitute this event.

TOAST OR TORTILLAS?

This program recommends toasted bread. The toast can be changed for corn tortillas toasted without oil. Each ounce of toast must be changed for one ounce of toasted tortilla. In my experience, fat loss is faster with corn tortillas. I recommend that you use them whenever you can obtain them.

It is possible that certain foods in the menus are not to your taste, or you may find some simply impossible to eat. Perhaps in certain seasons of the year you will not always find specific fruits marked in the menu. Or you could be allergic to some elements of the program, such as avocados, almonds, pecans, fish, etc. In these cases, you must carefully review the rations list presented in Appendix A of this book. With this list, you can make substitutions according to needs. For example, if you have an avocado allergy, replace the avocado with the indicated amount of olive or corn oil. If you don't like beans, you can change them for lentils, and so on. To avoid boredom, you can exchange one element on the menu for a different element in the same food group.

I love to recommend roasted almonds, but if you want to, you can easily substitute them for pistachios or cashews; eight roasted almonds equal eight cashews or twelve pistachios. You can also use pecans: for every almond you must eat one pecan half.

Distribute marked meals as evenly as possible throughout the day. If you establish a tight schedule, you will lose fat faster. If you wake up and go to sleep at the same time each day, you will also notice better results. You can also change food schedules. For example, dinner can be moved to lunchtime, and vice versa. But before modifying the menu, follow it as closely as possible for two consecutive weeks. By the third week, once you have learned how the program works, you can be more flexible in applying it.

Vegetables can be freely interchanges and I strongly recommend that you select the largest variety possible. Also remember that green leaf vegetables may favor loss of the waistline.

FAMILY AFFAIRS

Monday's menu of week three is similar to Monday's menu of weeks four, five, six, and seven. The major difference is that greater quantities are added each week to increase the number of calories. The same thing happens with the menus for other days of the week.

This way, the same meal can be prepared for the whole family, although quantities that each member eats may vary and each one can select the amount suited to his or her special needs. For example, men will surely feel better with quantities recommended for weeks five, six, or seven, while women perhaps will feel more satisfied with quantities recommended for weeks three and four.

Even if your family members are skinny, remember that all recommendations of the Bolio System comply with standard nutritional criteria, including those of the National Health Institute, American Heart Association, the American Cancer Society, and the American Diabetes Association for general healthy population. Rest assured that these programs are very healthy for any member of your family.

Your naturally skinny family members will also observe that any small excess of body fat will magically disappear. They may even observe how their glutei become more aesthetic and their body becomes more marked and athletic. Just don't be jealous of their results since those who have never dieted will usually obtain fast and spectacular changes with this program.

ROOM FOR VARIETY

There are thousands of foods and possible combinations that make eating a fascinating event. This program has tried to include plates preferred by the general American public, such as pancakes, cereals, biscuits, sandwiches, hamburgers, pizzas, etc.

But can a program be prepared with tofu, sausage, falafel, gumbo, clam chowder, lobsters, egg foo yung, sushi, quiche, ready to eat meals, or any other plate? The answer is yes, definitely, since there is no such thing as a forbidden plate in the Bolio System.

I will insist that you apply the program just as it is, without any major changes during at least twelve weeks. Once you have learned to enjoy a balanced and abundant meal, you can advance to enjoying a balanced, abundant and **varied** program.

The only rule that must always be covered in the Bolio System is that **the menu be balanced and sufficient.**

We can integrate any plate into the program, be it a personal recipe, a meal bought at the supermarket, or a special plate eaten at your favorite restaurant. If you are interested in this possibility, please contact us through the Internet:

www.drbolio.com (English version)
www.esbelto.com (Spanish version)

MONDAY

Early Morning Snack:	pineapple	1 cup
	almonds, roasted	6 each

Breakfast:	pancake or waffle	4 oz
	non fat milk, w/ vitamin A	8 fl oz

Mid-Morning Snack:	melon	1 cup
	almonds, roasted	6 each

Lunch:	toast	1 oz
	regular cottage cheese	2 oz
	mixed green salad	1 cup

Mid-Afternoon Snack:	watermelon	1 cup
	almonds, roasted	4 each

Dinner:	vegetable soup, no added fat	1 bowl
	tuna, canned in oil, drained	2 oz
	mayonnaise, regular	1 tbsp.
	mixed green salad	1 cup

Late Evening Snack:	honeydew melon	1 cup
	almonds, roasted	4 each

TUESDAY

Early Morning Snack:	watermelon	1 cup
	almonds, roasted	6 each

Breakfast:	plain non-fat yogurt	8 fl oz
	almonds, roasted	6 each
	papaya	1 cup
	honey	1 tbsp.

Mid-Morning Snack:	General Mills Total® whole grain cereal	1 cup
	almonds, roasted	4 each

Lunch:	black beans, boiled	½ cup
	mixed green salad	1 cup
	olive oil	2 tsp.
	toast	1 oz
	fruit juice w/ vitamin D	4 fl oz

Mid-Afternoon Snack:	mixed salad greens	1 cup
	sunflower oil	1 tsp.

Dinner:	skinless chicken breast	2 oz
	spaghetti, cooked (no fat)	½ cup
	mixed green salad	1 cup
	sunflower oil	1 tsp.

Late Evening Snack:	melon	1 cup
	almonds, roasted	4 each

WEDNESDAY

Early Morning Snack:	papaya	1 cup
	almonds, roasted	6 each

Breakfast:	biscuit, plain or buttermilk	2 oz
	non fat milk, w/ vitamin A	8 fl oz
	honey	1 tbsp.

Mid-Morning Snack:	banana, medium	1 each
	almonds, roasted	4 each

Lunch:	Sandwich:	
	mozzarella cheese	2 oz
	whole grain bread	2 oz (2 slices)
	tomato, onion, lettuce	free quantities
	fruit juice w/ vitamin D	6 fl oz

Mid-Afternoon Snack:	pineapple	1 cup
	almonds, roasted	4 each

Dinner:	beef, top round, lean	2 oz
	mixed green salad	1 cup
	sunflower oil	1 tsp.

Late Evening Snack:	melon	1 cup
	almonds, roasted	4 each

THURSDAY

Early Morning Snack:	watermelon	1 cup
	almonds, roasted	4 each

Breakfast:	non fat milk, w/ vitamin A	8 fl oz
	Kellogg's Complete® wheat bran flakes cereal	1 cup
	almonds, roasted	8 each

Mid-Morning Snack:	Swiss cheese	1 oz
	toast	1 oz

Lunch:	red kidney beans, boiled	½ cup
	vegetables, all types	1 cup
	olive oil	2 tsp.
	toast	1 regular slice
	fruit juice w/ vitamin D	6 fl oz

Mid-Afternoon Snack:	toast	1 oz
	honey	1 tbsp.

Dinner:	fish, steamed	3 oz
	white rice, cooked	½ cup
	mixed green salad	1 cup
	sunflower oil w/ vitamin E	1 tsp.

Late Evening Snack:	honeydew melon	1 cup
	almonds, roasted	4 each

FRIDAY

Early Morning Snack:	banana, medium	½ each
	almonds, roasted	4 each
	honey	1 tsp.

Breakfast:	egg, large	1 each
	egg white	1 oz
	tomato and onion	½ cup
	olive oil	1 tsp.
	fruit juice w/ vitamin D	4 fl oz

Mid-Morning Snack:	figs, dried, uncooked	2 each
	almonds, roasted	4 each

Lunch:	vegetable soup, no added fat	1 bowl
	chickpeas, cooked	½ cup
	whole grain bread	1 oz
	mixed salad greens	1 cup
	sunflower oil w/ vitamin E	1 tsp.

Mid-Afternoon Snack:	pear, medium	1 each
	almonds, roasted	4 each

Dinner:	salmon, cooked	4 oz
	vegetables, all types	1 cup
	white rice, cooked	½ cup
	whole grain bread	1 oz

Late Evening Snack:	ice cream	½ cup
	banana, medium	½ each

SATURDAY

Early Morning Snack:	grapefruit, medium	1 each
Breakfast:	melon	1 cup
	regular cottage cheese	½ cup
Mid-Morning Snack:	orange, medium	1 each
Lunch:	medium hamburger w/o mayonnaise (McDonald's Big n' Tasty®)	1 each
	side salad	1 serving
	small French fries	1 serving
	soft drink	16 fl oz
Mid-Afternoon Snack:	green-leaf salad	1 cup
	whole grain bread	1 oz
	tuna, canned in oil, drained	2 oz
Dinner:	Free (**but eat small portions**)	
Late Evening Snack:	papaya	1 cup

SUNDAY

Early Morning Snack:	watermelon	1 cup
Breakfast:	medium croissant	2 oz
	Swiss cheese	1 oz
	non fat milk, w/ vitamin A	6 fl oz
Mid-Morning Snack:	papaya	1 cup
Lunch:	cheese pizza	5 oz
	green-leaf salad	1 cup
	fruit juice w/ vitamin D	8 fl oz
Mid-Afternoon Snack:	popcorn, popped in oil	3 cups
Dinner:	General Mills Total* whole grain cereal	1 cup
	non fat milk, w/ vitamin A	8 fl oz
Late Evening Snack:	melon	1 cup

Week Four

MONDAY

Early Morning Snack:	pineapple	1 cup
	almonds, roasted	6 each
Breakfast:	pancake or waffle	4 oz
	non fat milk, w/ vitamin A	8 fl oz
	maple syrup	5 tsp
	butter	2 tsp.
Mid-Morning Snack:	melon	1 cup
	almonds, roasted	6 each
Lunch:	toast	2 oz
	regular cottage cheese	2 oz
	lettuce, raw	1 cup
Mid-Afternoon Snack:	watermelon	1 cup
	almonds, roasted	4 each
Dinner:	vegetable soup, w/o fat	1 bowl
	tuna, canned in oil, drained	4 oz
	mayonnaise, regular	1 tbsp.
	vegetables, all types	1 cup
Late Evening Snack:	honeydew melon	1 cup
	almonds, roasted	4 each

TUESDAY

Early Morning Snack:	watermelon	1 cup
	almonds, roasted	4 each

Breakfast:	plain non-fat yogurt	8 fl oz
	almonds, roasted	8 each
	papaya	1 cup
	honey	1 tbsp.

Mid-Morning Snack:	General Mills Total® whole grain cereal	1 cup
	almonds, roasted	6 each

Lunch:	black beans, boiled	½ cup
	olive oil	2 tsp.
	vegetables, all types	1 cup
	whole grain bread	1 oz
	fruit juice w/ vitamin D	6 fl oz

Mid-Afternoon Snack:	green leaf salad	1 cup
	sunflower oil	2 tsp.

Dinner:	roasted chicken breast w/o skin	2 oz
	spaghetti, cooked w/o oil	½ cup
	mixed green salad	1 cup
	sunflower oil	2 tsp.
	fruit juice w/ vitamin D	6 fl oz

Late Evening Snack:	melon	1 cup
	almonds, roasted	4 each

WEDNESDAY

Early Morning Snack:	apple, medium	1 each
	almonds, roasted	6 each
Breakfast:	biscuit, plain or buttermilk	2 oz
	honey	1 tbsp.
	non fat milk, w/ vitamin A	8 fl oz
Mid-Morning Snack:	banana, medium	1 each
	almonds, roasted	6 each
Lunch:	Sandwich:	
	Mozzarella cheese	2 oz
	Wheat bread	2 oz
	mayonnaise, regular	2 tsp.
	Tomato, onion, lettuce	free quantities
	fruit juice w/ vitamin D	8 fl oz
Mid-Afternoon Snack:	pineapple	1 cup
	almonds, roasted	4 each
Dinner:	beef, top round, lean	2 oz
	mixed green salad	1 cup
	sunflower oil	1 tsp.
	whole grain bread	1 oz
Late Evening Snack:	melon	1 cup
	almonds, roasted	4 each

THURSDAY

Early Morning Snack:	watermelon	1 cup
	almonds, roasted	6 each

Breakfast:	non fat milk, w/ vitamin A	8 fl oz
	Kellogg's Complete® wheat bran flakes cereal	1 cup
	almonds, roasted	8 each
	fruit juice w/ vitamin D	5 fl oz

Mid-Morning Snack:	Swiss cheese	1 oz
	toast	1 oz
	honey	1 tbsp.

Lunch:	red kidney beans, cooked	½ cup
	vegetables, all types	1 cup
	olive oil	2 tsp.
	toast	1 oz
	fruit juice w/ vitamin D	5 fl oz

Mid-Afternoon Snack:	toast	1 oz
	honey	1 tsp.

Dinner:	steamed fish	4 oz
	white rice, cooked	½ cup
	vegetables, all types	1 cup
	sunflower oil w/vitamin E	2 tsp.

Late Evening Snack:	melon	1 cup
	almonds, roasted	4 each

FRIDAY

Early Morning Snack:	banana, medium	½ each
	almonds, roasted	4 each
	honey	1 tbsp.

Breakfast:	egg, large	1 each
	egg white	1 oz
	tomato and onion	½ cup
	olive oil	1 tsp.
	fruit juice w/ vitamin D	8 fl oz

Mid-Morning Snack:	figs, dried, uncooked	2 each
	almonds, roasted	6 each

Lunch:	vegetable soup, no added fat	1 bowl
	chickpeas, cooked	½ cup
	whole grain bread	1 oz
	mixed greens salad	1 cup
	sunflower oil w/vitamin E	2 tsp.

Mid-Afternoon Snack:	pear, medium	1 each
	almonds, roasted	6 each

Dinner:	salmon, cooked	4 oz
	vegetables, all types	1 cup
	white rice, cooked	1 cup

Late Evening Snack:	ice cream, any flavor	½ cup
	banana, medium	½ each

SATURDAY

Early Morning Snack:	grapefruit	1 each
Breakfast:	regular cottage cheese	½ cup
	melon	1 cup
	almonds, roasted	6 each
	fruit juice w/ vitamin D	4 fl oz
Mid-Morning Snack:	orange, medium	1 each
	almonds, roasted	4 each
Lunch:	medium hamburger w/o mayonnaise (Mc Donald's Big 'n Tasty®)	1 each
	side salad	1 serving
	small French fries	1 serving
	soft drink	16 fl oz
Mid-Afternoon Snack:	mixed greens salad	1 cup
	whole grain bread	1 oz
	tuna, canned in oil, drained	2 oz
Dinner:	Free **(but eat small portions)**	
Late Evening Snack:	apple, medium	1 each
	almonds, roasted	4 each

SUNDAY

Early Morning Snack:	watermelon	1 cup
Breakfast:	medium croissant	1 each
	Swiss cheese	1 oz
	non fat milk, w/ vitamin A	8 fl oz
	fruit juice w/ vitamin D	5 fl oz
Mid-Morning Snack:	pear, medium	1 each
Lunch:	cheese pizza	6 oz
	green-leaf salad	1 cup
Mid-Afternoon Snack:	popcorn popped in oil	4 cups
Dinner:	General Mills Total® whole grain cereal	1 cup
	non fat milk, w/ vitamin A	8 fl oz
Late Evening Snack:	melon	1 cup
	almonds, roasted	4 each

Week Five

MONDAY

Early Morning Snack:	banana, medium	1 each
	almonds, roasted	6 each
Breakfast:	pancake or waffle	4 oz
	non fat milk, w/ vitamin A	8 fl oz
	maple syrup	4 tsp
	butter	1 tsp.
Mid-Morning Snack:	apple, medium	1 each
	almonds, roasted	6 each
Lunch:	toast	2 oz
	regular cottage cheese	½ cup
	mixed salad greens, raw	1 cup
	fruit juice w/ vitamin D	5 fl oz
Mid-Afternoon Snack:	watermelon	1 cup
	almonds, roasted	4 each
Dinner:	vegetable soup, no added fat	1 bowl
	tuna, canned in oil, drained	2 oz
	mayonnaise	1 tbsp.
	crackers	½ oz
	mixed salad greens, raw	1 cup
Late Evening Snack:	melon	1 cup
	almonds, roasted	6 each

TUESDAY

Early Morning Snack:	banana	1 each
	almonds, roasted halves	4 each

Breakfast:	plain non-fat yogurt	8 fl oz
	almonds, roasted	8 each
	papaya	1 cup
	honey	1 tbsp.

Mid-Morning Snack:	Sandwich:	2 oz
	whole grain bread	
	turkey breast, fat free	1 oz
	mayonnaise	2 tsp.
	fruit juice w/ vitamin D	6 fl oz

Lunch:	black beans, boiled	½ cup
	vegetables, all types	1 cup
	olive oil	2 tsp.
	whole grain bread	1 oz
	fruit juice w/ vitamin D	8 fl oz

Mid-Afternoon Snack:	mixed salad, greens, raw	1 cup
	sunflower oil w/ vitamin E	2 tsp.

Dinner:	skinless chicken breast	2 oz
	spaghetti, cooked w/o oil	½ cup
	mixed salad greens, raw	1 cup
	sunflower oil w/ vitamin E	2 tsp.

Late Evening Snack:	melon	1 cup
	almonds, roasted	4 each

WEDNESDAY

Early Morning Snack:	apple, medium	1 each
	almonds, roasted	6 each

Breakfast:	biscuit, plain or buttermilk	4 oz
	non-fat milk w/ vitamin A	8 fl oz
	honey	1 tbsp.

Mid-Morning Snack:	pineapple	1 cup
	almonds, roasted	6 each

Lunch:	Sandwich:	
	mozzarella cheese	2 oz
	wheat bread	2 oz (2 slices)
	mayonnaise	2 tsp.
	tomato, onion, lettuce	free quantities
	fruit juice w/ vitamin D	8 fl oz

Mid-Afternoon Snack:	pineapple	1 cup
	almonds, roasted	4 each

Dinner:	beef, top round, lean	2 oz
	white rice, boiled	½ cup
	vegetables, all types	1 cup
	sunflower oil w/ vitamin E	1 tsp.

Late Evening Snack:	melon	1 cup
	almonds, roasted	4 each

THURSDAY

Early Morning Snack:	apple, medium	1 each
	almonds, roasted	6 each

Breakfast:	non-fat milk, w/ vitamin A	8 fl oz
	Kellogg's Complete® wheat bran flakes cereal	1 cup
	almonds, roasted	8 each

Mid-Morning Snack:	Swiss cheese	1 oz
	toast	1 oz
	honey	1 tbsp.

Lunch:	toast	2 oz
	Mixed salad greens, raw	1 cup
	red kidney beans, cooked	½ cup
	olive oil	2 tsp.
	fruit juice w/ vitamin D	8 fl oz

Mid-Afternoon Snack:	toast	1 oz
	butter	1 tsp.
	honey	1 tbsp.

Dinner:	fish, steamed	4 oz
	white rice, cooked	½ cup
	mixed salad greens	1 cup
	sunflower oil w/ vitamin E	2 tsp.

Late Evening Snack:	pear, medium	1 each
	almonds, roasted	4 each

FRIDAY

Early Morning Snack:	banana	½ each
	almonds, roasted	6 each
	honey	1 tbsp.

Breakfast:	egg, large	1 each
	egg white	1 oz
	tomato and onion	½ cup
	olive oil	2 tsp.
	whole grain bread	1 oz
	fruit juice w/ vitamin D	8 fl. oz

Mid-Morning Snack:	figs, dried, uncooked	2 each
	almonds, roasted	6 each

Lunch:	vegetable soup, w/o fat	1 bowl
	chickpeas, cooked	½ cup
	turkey breast	2 oz
	mixed salad greens, raw	1 cup
	sunflower oil w/ vitamin E	1 tsp.
	fruit juice w/ vitamin D	8 fl oz.

Mid-Afternoon Snack:	pear, medium	1 each
	almonds, roasted	6 each

Dinner:	salmon, cooked	4 oz
	white rice, cooked	1 cup
	mixed salad greens, raw	1 cup
	sunflower oil w/ vitamin E	1 tsp.

Late Evening Snack:	ice cream	½ cup
	banana	½ each

SATURDAY

Early Morning Snack:	grapefruit, medium	1 each

Breakfast:	regular cottage cheese	1 cup
	melon	1 cup
	almonds, roasted	4 each
	All Bran cereal	½ cup
	fruit juice w/ vitamin D	6 fl oz

Mid-Morning Snack:	orange, medium	1 each
	almonds, roasted	4 each

Lunch:	medium hamburger w/o mayonnaise (McDonald's Big n' Tasty®)	1 each
	side salad	1 serving
	small French fries	1 serving
	soft drink	16 fl oz

Mid-Afternoon Snack:	green-leaf salad	1 cup
	whole grain bread	1 oz
	tuna, canned in oil, drained	2 oz

Dinner:	Free (**but eat small portions**)	

Late Evening Snack:	apple, medium	1 each
	almonds, roasted	4 each

SUNDAY

Early Morning Snack:	watermelon	1 cup
	almonds, roasted	4 each

Breakfast:	croissant, medium	1 each
	American cheese, non fat, Kraft	2 oz
	non-fat milk, w/ vitamin A	8 fl oz
	fruit juice w/ vitamin D	8 fl oz

Mid-Morning Snack:	pear, medium	1 each
	Almonds, roasted	4 each

Lunch:	cheese pizza	6 oz
	green-leaf salad	1 cup
	fruit juice w/ vitamin D	8 fl oz

Mid-Afternoon Snack:	popcorn popped in oil	4 cups

Dinner:	General Mills Total® whole grain cereal	1 cup
	non-fat milk w/ vitamin A	8 fl oz
	almonds, roasted	6 each

Late Evening Snack:	melon	1 cup
	almonds, roasted	4 each

Week Six

MONDAY

Early Morning Snack:	banana, medium	1 each
	almonds, roasted	4 each

Breakfast:	pancake or waffle	4 oz
	non-fat milk w/ vitamin A	8 fl oz
	maple syrup	1 tbsp
	butter	2 tsp.

Mid-Morning Snack:	papaya	1 cup
	almonds, roasted	4 each

Lunch:	toast	1 oz
	regular cottage cheese	4 oz
	vegetables, all types	1 cup
	fruit juice w/ vitamin D	8 fl. oz.

Mid-Afternoon Snack:	glazed doughnut	2 oz

Dinner:	vegetable soup, w/o fat	1 bowl
	tuna, canned in oil, drained	4 oz
	crackers	½ oz
	mixed salad greens, raw	1 cup

Late Evening Snack:	melon	1 cup
	almonds, roasted	4 each

TUESDAY

Early Morning Snack:	banana	1 each
	almonds, roasted halves	6 each

Breakfast:	plain non-fat yogurt	8 fl oz
	almonds, roasted	8 each
	papaya	1 cup
	honey	1 tbsp.

Mid-Morning Snack:	Sandwich:	
	whole grain bread	2 oz
	turkey breast	1 oz
	mayonnaise	2 tsp.
	fruit juice w/ vitamin D	8 fl oz

Lunch:	black beans, boiled	½ cup
	vegetables, all types	1 cup
	olive oil	2 tsp.
	wheat bread	1 oz
	fruit juice w/ vitamin D	8 fl oz

Mid-Afternoon Snack:	apple pie, two crusts	2 oz

Dinner:	skinless chicken breast	4 oz
	spaghetti, cooked w/o oil	½ cup
	mixed salad greens, raw	1 cup
	sunflower oil w/ vitamin E	2 tsp.

Late Evening Snack:	melon	1 cup
	almonds, roasted	6 each

WEDNESDAY

| Early Morning Snack: | apple, medium | 1 each |
| | almonds, roasted | 6 each |

Breakfast:	biscuit, plain or buttermilk	4 oz
	non-fat milk w/ vitamin A	8 fl oz
	honey	1 tbsp.

| Mid-Morning Snack: | banana, medium | 1 each |
| | almonds, roasted | 4 each |

Lunch:	Sandwich:	
	mozzarella cheese	1 oz
	wheat bread	2 oz
	tomato, onion, lettuce	free quantities
	fruit juice w/ vitamin D	8 fl oz

| Mid-Afternoon Snack: | chocolate pound cake | 2 oz |

Dinner:	beef, top round, lean	4 oz
	vegetables, all types	1 cup
	sunflower oil w/ vitamin E	2 tsp.
	white rice, cooked w/o oil	½ cup

| Late Evening Snack: | melon | 1 cup |
| | almonds, roasted | 6 each |

THURSDAY

Early Morning Snack:	apple, medium	1 each
	almonds, roasted	4 each
Breakfast:	non-fat milk w/ vitamin A	8 fl oz
	Kellogg's Complete Wheat bran flakes cereal	
	almonds, roasted	4 each
	fruit juice w/ vitamin D	8 fl oz
Mid-Morning Snack:	Swiss cheese	1 oz
	toast	1 oz
	honey	1 tbsp.
Lunch:	toast	1 oz
	vegetables, all types	1 cup
	small red beans	½ cup
	Swiss cheese	2 oz
	olive oil	2 tsp.
	fruit juice w/ vitamin D	8 fl oz
Mid-Afternoon Snack:	coffee cake	2 oz
Dinner:	steamed fish	4 oz
	white rice, cooked	½ cup
	vegetables, all types	1 cup
	sunflower oil w/ vitamin E	2 tsp.
Late Evening Snack:	pear, medium	1 each
	almonds, roasted	5 each

FRIDAY

Early Morning Snack:	banana, medium	½ each
	almonds, roasted	4 each
	honey	1 tbsp.

Breakfast:	egg, large	1 each
	egg white	1 oz
	tomato and onion	½ cup
	olive oil	1 tsp.
	whole grain bread	2 oz
	fruit juice w/ vitamin D	8 fl oz

Mid-Morning Snack:	figs, dried, uncooked	2 each
	almonds, roasted	4 each

Lunch:	vegetable soup, w/o fat	1 bowl
	Lentils, cooked	½ cup
	turkey breast	1 oz
	mixed salad greens	1 cup
	sunflower oil w/ vitamin E	1 tsp.
	whole grain bread	2 oz

Mid-Afternoon Snack:	cheesecake	4 oz

Dinner:	salmon, cooked	4 oz
	rice, cooked	1 cup
	vegetables, all types	1 cup
	sunflower oil w/ vitamin E	1 tsp.

Late Evening Snack:	ice cream	½ cup
	banana	½ each

SATURDAY

Early Morning Snack:	grapefruit, medium	1 each
	sugar, brown or white	1 tsp.

Breakfast:	regular cottage cheese	1 cup
	almonds, roasted halves	8 each
	melon	1 cup
	All Bran cereal	½ cup
	fruit juice w/ vitamin D	8 fl oz

Mid-Morning Snack:	orange, medium	1 each
	almonds, roasted	4 each

Lunch:	medium hamburger w/o mayonnaise (McDonald's Big n' Tasty®)	1 each
	side salad	1 serving
	small French fries	1 serving
	soft drink	16 fl oz

Mid-Afternoon Snack:	mixed salad greens, raw	1 cup
	whole grain bread	2 oz
	tuna, canned in oil, drained	2 oz
	mayonnaise	2 tsp.

Dinner:	Free (but eat small portions)	

Late Evening Snack:	apple, medium	1 each
	almonds, roasted	4 each

SUNDAY

Early Morning Snack:	watermelon	1 cup
Breakfast:	croissant	2 oz
	American cheese, non fat, Kraft	2 slices
	non-fat milk w/ vitamin A	8 fl oz
	fruit juice w/ vitamin D	8 fl oz
Mid-Morning Snack:	pear, medium	1 each
Lunch:	meat pizza	6 oz
	green-leaf salad	1 cup
	fruit juice w/ vitamin D	8 fl oz
Mid-Afternoon Snack:	popcorn, popped in oil	6 cups
Dinner:	General Mills Total® Whole grain cereal	1 cup
	non-fat milk w/ vitamin A	8 fl oz
	almonds, roasted	6 each
Late Evening Snack:	melon	1 cup
	almonds	4 each

Week Seven

MONDAY

| Early Morning Snack: | banana, medium | 1 each |
| | almonds, roasted | 4 each |

Breakfast:	pancake or waffle	4 oz
	non-fat milk w/ vitamin A	8 fl oz
	maple syrup	1 tbsp.
	butter	2 tsp.

| Mid-Morning Snack: | apple, medium | 1 each |
| | almonds, roasted | 4 each |

Lunch:	toast	2 oz
	regular cottage cheese	4 oz
	mixed salad greens, raw	1 cup
	fruit juice w/ vitamin D	8 fl oz

| Mid-Afternoon Snack: | glazed doughnut | 4 oz |

Dinner:	vegetable soup, w/o fat	1 bowl
	tuna, canned in oil, drained	4 oz
	crackers	½ oz
	mixed salad greens, raw	1 cup

| Late Evening Snack: | melon | 1 cup |
| | almonds, roasted | 2 each |

TUESDAY

Early Morning Snack:	banana	1 each
	almonds, roasted halves	6 each

Breakfast:	plain non-fat yogurt	8 fl oz
	almonds, roasted	8 each
	All Bran® cereal	½ cup
	papaya	1 cup
	honey	1 tbsp.

Mid-Morning Snack:	Sandwich:	
	bread	2 oz
	turkey breast, fat free	1 oz
	mayonnaise	2 tsp.
	fruit juice w/ vitamin D	8 fl oz

Lunch:	black beans, boiled	½ cup
	vegetables, all types	1 cup
	olive oil	2 tsp.
	whole grain bread	1 oz
	fruit juice w/ vitamin D	8 fl oz

Mid-Afternoon Snack:	apple pie (two crusts)	4 oz

Dinner:	skinless chicken breast	4 oz
	cooked pasta	½ cup
	mixed salad greens, raw	1 cup
	sunflower oil w/ vitamin E	2 tsp.

Late Evening Snack:	melon	1 cup
	almonds, roasted	6 each

WEDNESDAY

Early Morning Snack:	melon	1 cup
	almonds, roasted	4 each

Breakfast:	biscuit, plain or buttermilk	4 oz
	non-fat milk w/ vitamin A	8 fl oz
	honey	1 tbsp.

Mid-Morning Snack:	banana, medium	1 each
	almonds, roasted	4 each

Lunch:	Sandwich:	
	non fat American cheese	2 oz
	ham	1 oz
	whole grain bread	2 oz
	tomato, onion, lettuce	free quantities
	fruit juice w/ vitamin D	8 fl oz

Mid-Afternoon Snack:	chocolate pound cake	4 oz

Dinner:	beef, top round, lean	4 oz
	cooked rice	½ cup
	mixed greens salad, raw	1 cup
	sunflower oil w/ vitamin E	1 tsp.

Late Evening Snack:	honeydew melon	1 cup
	almonds, roasted	4 each

THURSDAY

Early Morning Snack:	apple, medium	1 each
	almonds, roasted	6 each

Breakfast:	non-fat milk w/ vitamin A	8 fl oz
	Kellogg's Complete wheat bran flakes	1 cup
	almonds, roasted	8 each
	fruit juice w/ vitamin D	8 fl oz

Mid-Morning Snack:	Swiss cheese	1 oz
	toast	1 oz
	honey	4 tsp

Lunch:	toast	1 oz
	small red beans	½ cup
	Swiss cheese, low fat	2 oz
	Mixed salad greens, raw	1 cup
	olive oil	1 tsp.
	fruit juice w/ vitamin D	8 fl oz

Mid-Afternoon Snack:	chocolate pound cake	4 oz

Dinner:	steamed fish	4 oz
	white rice, cooked	½ cup
	vegetables, all types	1 cup
	sunflower oil w/ vitamin E	2 tsp.

Late Evening Snack:	pear, medium	1 each
	almonds, roasted	4 each

FRIDAY

Early Morning Snack:	banana	½ each
	almonds, roasted	6 each
	honey	1 tbsp.

Breakfast:	egg, large	1 each
	egg white	1 oz
	tomato and onion	½ cup
	olive oil	1 tsp.
	bread	1 oz
	fruit juice w/ vitamin D	8 fl oz

Mid-Morning Snack:	figs, dried, uncooked	3 each
	almonds, roasted	4 each

Lunch:	vegetable soup, no added fat	1 bowl
	chickpeas, cooked	½ cup
	ham	1 oz
	vegetables, all types	1 cup
	sunflower oil w/ vitamin E	1 tsp.
	bread	2 oz
	fruit juice w/ vitamin D	8 fl oz

Mid-Afternoon Snack:	cheesecake	4 oz

Dinner:	salmon, cooked	4 oz
	rice, cooked	1 cup
	mixed greens salad, raw	1 cup
	sunflower oil w/ vitamin E	1 tsp.

Late Evening Snack:	ice cream	½ cup
	banana	½ each

SATURDAY

Early Morning Snack:	grapefruit, medium	1 each
	sugar	1 tsp.
	almonds, roasted	6 each

Breakfast:	melon	1 cup
	regular cottage cheese	1 cup
	almonds, roasted	8 each
	Special K	½ cup

Mid-Morning Snack:	fruit	1 each
	almonds, roasted	4 each

Lunch:	medium hamburger w/o mayonnaise (McDonald's Big n' Tasty®)	1 each
	side salad	1 serving
	small French fries	1 serving
	soft drink	16 fl oz

Mid-Afternoon Snack:	green-leaf salad	1 cup
	bread	2 oz
	tuna, canned in oil, drained	4 oz
	fruit juice w/ vitamin D	8 fl oz

Dinner:	Free (but eat small portions)	

Late Evening Snack:	apple	1 each
	almonds, roasted halves	4 each

SUNDAY

Early Morning Snack:	watermelon	1 cup
	Almonds, roasted	4 each
Breakfast:	butter croissant	4 oz
	regular cottage cheese	1 cup
	non-fat milk w/ vitamin A	8 fl oz
Mid-Morning Snack:	pear, medium	1 each
Lunch:	cheese pizza	6 oz
	green-leaf salad	1 cup
	soft drink	16 fl oz
Mid-Afternoon Snack:	popcorn, popped in oil	5 cups
Dinner:	General Mills Total® whole grain cereal	1 cup
	non-fat milk w/ vitamin A	8 fl oz
	almonds, roasted	8 each
Late Evening Snack:	melon	1 cup
	almonds, roasted	4 each

Week Eight

No two human beings are truly identical. There always will be biological, social, and psychological differences. Food needs are no exception. Some require large quantities of food all during the day, since their physical activity is constant and intense. Others have busy mornings and calm evenings. Any change in energy needs is quickly detected by our brain, and appetite is reduced or increased accordingly.

In the rigid recommendations set out in weeks three to seven, portions are uniformly distributed throughout the day, thus generating a faster reduction of body fat. You must not eat less than is recommended, or you will run the risk of upsetting the balance in your diet and regaining all the body fat you have lost.

This lack of flexibility can perhaps lead to hunger in the morning and lack of appetite in the afternoon. Maybe breakfast is such a misery that you need to add extra shakes, and dinner seems more like martyrdom from overeating than a pleasant meal.

Food needs also change from day to day. Perhaps the dinner menu from Monday to Friday provides more than enough, but on Sunday you need much more than is recommended.

The only way to solve this is to eat without fear, listen to your body, and take at every moment of the day all that you need to feel satisfied.

The task now is to learn to eat freely while still following the central principles of the program. Only general recommendations will be given, and you will be responsible for deciding what you eat, how much you eat, and when you eat it. It is time to apply all that you have learned, and test yourself to see how many of your eating habits have changed.

How will you know that you are still eating a balanced meal?

Several studies that I carried out in the Mexican Institute of Social Security demonstrated a change in eating patterns four weeks after beginning this program. Those studied woke up hungry, wanted something to eat every two to three hours, ate more fruits and vegetables, and spontaneously reduced their consumption of fats. No participant was conscious of these changes. Those studied had begun to spontaneously eat a balanced diet. What was the final result? They spontaneously began to eat a balanced meal.

If you have followed recommendations of the Bolio System to this point, your body will now surely notify you through appetite and satiety what to eat in order to achieve nutritional balance.

Don't fool yourself into thinking that you can control the way you eat for the rest of your life. This makes no sense, since our brains have been telling us for millions of years exactly what to eat to stay naturally thin. Don't be afraid that your brain cells might have been damaged by too many diets or that they have permanently fallen asleep. We don't pay any attention to our natural instincts simply because we are afraid that food will make us fat.

The great paradox of those with excess body fat is that to eliminate their problem, they must do exactly what they have always avoided; give their body what it asks for.

In this week, you must try to eliminate forever the bad habit of rationing and restricting what you eat. Not until you allow your body to establish what, when, and how much to eat will you be able to eradicate excess body fat. So let's get to work. It is time to let your body take control of your eating habits.

MAINTENANCE PLAN

EARLY MORNING SNACK:

Eat one of the following:

- a shake (see Recovery Phase of week one)
- fresh fruit and/or fruit juice with nuts
- regular yogurt, any flavor

BREAKFAST:

Eat fresh fruit and/or fruit juice plus one of the following options:

- Any type of processed cereal, such as Corn Flakes or Captain Crunch; non-fat milk; almonds, roasted or cashews

- Bagel with low fat crème cheese

- Biscuit with 1% fat milk

- Boiled beans or lentils; vegetables; olive oil or avocado; whole grain bread

- Corn or flour tortillas with lean steak or chicken breast or low fat cheese

- Croissant with turkey breast or low fat ham or low fat cheese

- Eggs cooked in olive oil (maximum of two times per week); vegetables; boiled beans; whole grain bread.

- Hot dog

- Pancakes or waffles with butter plus honey or maple syrup and non-fat milk.

- Pastry with non-fat milk

- Sandwich with whole grain bread and turkey, ham, low-fat cheese, tuna, or sardines; olive oil or avocado; tomatoes and/or onions

- Toasted corn tortillas or bread toast with beans, avocado and green leaf vegetables

    (Any of these recommendations, except for the scrambled eggs, can be taken as breakfast, lunch, or dinner. Quantities are left to the judgment of each person.)

MID-MORNING SNACK:

Eat one of the following:

- Fresh fruit, dried fruit and/or fruit juice with nuts
- Almonds, cashews, or any other nut
- Regular yogurt, any flavor
- Cereal bars (Granola, etc.)
- Crackers
- Coffee or tea with brown sugar
- A shake (see Recovery Phase of week one)
- Any of the recommendations marked for breakfast

LUNCH:

Eat any of the recommendations for breakfast or one of the following:

- Beans, lentils, or chickpeas with olive oil, vegetables, bread and fruit juice
- 1 medium hamburger with green leaf salad and fruit juice
- 1 medium pizza with green leaf salad and fruit juice
- Chicken, fish or beef with vegetables, bread and fruit juice

MID-AFTERNOON SNACK:

Eat any of the recommendations for the mid-morning snack.

DINNER:

Any type of soup prepared without oil; boiled rice or pasta; raw or cooked vegetables; beans, lentils, or any other legume; meat, chicken, or fish; any type of bread; non-diet soft drink or fruit juice; olive oil, any type of salad dressing or avocado; almonds, or cashews; any type of dessert such as apple pie, chocolate chip cookies, etc.

LATE EVENING SNACK:

Eat one of the following:

- A shake (see Recovery Phase of week one)
- Fresh fruit or fruit juice
- Ice cream
- Regular yogurt, any flavor
- Whole milk

EARLY MORNING SNACK:

Try to maintain the habit of eating immediately after opening your eyes.

Have something low in calories, but if your body needs more, exchange the yogurt or fresh fruit for a piece of apple pie or even the shake indicated in week one. Remember to eat this small portion of food before any another activity, such as taking a shower or undertaking any physical activity. Who decides how much to eat? You do.

BREAKFAST:

Have fresh fruit and/or fruit juice plus any of the options recommended for breakfast.

If you are 30 or older, eat a maximum of two egg yolks per week. If you are eating more and know through laboratory tests that your blood cholesterol is normal, you may have eggs up to four times a week if your doctor allows it.

You can prepare your sandwich with any type of bread such as baguette, pita bread, etc.

Any of the other options may be eaten at any moment of the day. A sandwich and/or pancakes can be taken at mid-morning, at mid-afternoon, or late at night as supper. Who decides what and how much to eat? It's your body's decision.

MID-MORNING SNACK:

Select a plate that is easy to prepare and transport.

If you have the desire and the opportunity, eat any of the breakfast recommendations. But if your lifestyle is very hectic, don't try any of these more elaborate options for your snack. It will only distress you instead of making you skinny.

From a metabolic point of view, the best option for a mid-morning snack is a sandwich. But it is wiser to follow a practical nutritional plan than to overwhelm your already burdened life with options that force you to load up your purse or briefcase with food.

Perhaps your job does not allow you to eat a sandwich. In this case, have fruit juice, dried fruit, crackers, a shake, and/or regular yogurt with fruit.

LUNCH:

Select any of the listed options. But be very careful when repeating any particular option or you may end up eating a boring diet. Of course, if you are a sandwich or hamburger addict, have as many as you want; you will still lose excess fat. When I want patients to quickly lose weight, I usually recommend a diet based on sandwiches.

According to many studies, the human body's response to food (thermogenesis) is more efficient during the early hours of the day and is curtailed by late afternoon. Therefore, it is wise to eat a good breakfast, a hearty lunch, and a very small dinner.

This does not mean that you must eat this way to stay slender. If you have a small lunch and a hearty dinner, continue with this habit and test the results with your measuring tape. If you observe a satisfactory reduction of weight and inches, continue with your usual eating pattern. But if you see no change, add more food to your lunch.

MID-AFTERNOON SNACK:

Select any of the options recommended for breakfast or the mid-morning snack, but be careful of quantities, or you may end up overly full by the end of the third day of this week. This can lead you to react by eating too little food, resulting in malnutrition and finally further accumulation of body fat.

DINNER:

Eat everything that is recommended: any kind of soup that contains vegetables; boiled rice or pasta; legumes such as beans or lentils; raw and/or cooked vegetables; protein from meat, chicken, fish, or seafood; fats from avocados, nuts, and/or olive oil; cereals such as bread or corn tortillas; refined sugar such as your favorite soft drink or fruit juice; and finally any type of dessert.

Many complain that they are not able to eat all of the recommended items. Start with small portions, and gradually increase them until you find the proper quantities. Eat everything that is recommended, even if it is only a minimal amount, or you will run the risk of preparing an unbalanced meal.

If you are so hungry that you need to repeat the dinner menu two, three, or four times a day, there is no problem. Just make sure that you eat at least seven times a day; if you ate a hearty dinner and still feel full before going to sleep, you must still eat something, even though you are not hungry. In traditional diets, you cannot eat extra quantities when you're hungry. In this program, you must eat at least seven times a day even when you are not hungry.

LATE EVENING SNACK:

Some people have dinner and immediately go to sleep. If you do this, don't worry. This eating pattern will not result in an accumulation of body fat.

Other people have a very small and early dinner and do not go to sleep until several hours later. If this is your custom, have two or more small snacks before going to sleep. This way, you will reduce fasting to a minimum.

A small amount of fruit before going to sleep is more than enough for most of us. But if you want ice cream or chocolate bars, go ahead. Other things you can include are: any type of pastry, whole milk, regular yogurt, strawberries with cream, and crackers with butter.

When you eat carbohydrates associated with fats before going to sleep, insulin requirements for next day's breakfast are reduced, thus favoring the loss of body fat. This is even true for diabetics, but a word of caution, add these types of foods to your evening **only with your doctor's knowledge and consent**.

Sounds great, right? Science has found new and pleasant ways to reduce excess body fat. But you will not achieve this as long as you fear food.

EATING MANY TIMES A DAY

There are many advantages to eating frequently during the day.

In first place, this practice reduces prolonged fasting. Remember that, according to the many studies cited in previous chapters, prolonged and continuous fasting promotes the accumulation of body fat.

Second, when you eat many times a day, your body's thermogenic response is increased. In non-medical terms, this means that your body will more easily turn excess food into heat instead of body fat.

Third, and this is most important in the battle to change eating patterns, when you eat more often, you automatically and unconsciously modify the way you eat.

You can very easily demonstrate this response; select your most addictive food group, apple pies, chocolate bars or any other "addictive" food. Divide your favorite and addictive food into small fractions, in such a way that you can eat every hour without causing nausea. By the fifth or sixth helping, you will note a desire to change your plate for some other food group. You will also notice that after the sixth helping, you will spontaneously reduce the amount needed to feel satisfied.

When giving lectures, I enjoy recommending that people eat whatever they want as long as they do it every one to two hours. By the third day, they usually notice that their measurements have decreased, even though they are eating their favorite food, no matter what it is. This way, they quickly understand that the way they eat is more important than what and how much they eat.

Fourth, every time we eat, it increases the general activity of our body (our basal metabolism).

If you have not acquired the habit of eating frequently by now, you run the risk of quickly losing interest in following the Bolio System. You may even stop having some food group and end up accumulating body fat through an unbalanced diet. To prevent this, start with small-to-moderate portions. If, after three days, you realize that you can eat more without feeling full, go ahead and have larger quantities. This program contains all the necessary elements for a satisfactory and slow reduction of weight and inches.

Be very attentive to your body's needs. If you desire a particular food group not listed on the menus, go ahead and eat it .Why? Because your brain is telling you that it requires other elements. But always keep in mind the prudent recommendation of eating small portions of saturated fats.

DIETARY FAT

Sometimes it is difficult to establish optimum quantities of dietary fat. Those who learn that fats are responsible for excess body fat lose their fear of carbohydrates but sometimes develop an unhealthy fear of animal and vegetable fats. Fear of becoming overweight does not allow them to listen to their bodies, and, just in case, they decide to limit their intake of fats. This can be counteractive, since a very low-fat diet may lead to regaining the weight and inches already lost.

Is there a way to know exactly when you are taking insufficient amounts of fats?

There is no quick and direct way to establish that you have been too stingy with your fat rations. But your body does present changes that you can identify, and if they do appear, you must quickly make appropriate changes to your diet.

If your hair becomes brittle and without shine, and if your skin is dry (in spite of smearing on jars of costly creams), it could be that you are not eating enough fats. Vegetable oils increase beauty because they favor a silky shiny hair and smooth skin.

If you have frequent infections of the respiratory or genital tract, you may have suppressed your immune system through inadequate oil consumption. Besides going to your doctor, increase vegetable fats in your menu.

If you recognize any of these signs, add more nuts, avocado, chocolate and/or any other vegetable fat to your menu until signs disappear. You will observe how respiratory infections subside and your hair becomes silkier in spite of torturing it with various chemical products.

REPEATING WEEK EIGHT

You can continue with week eight as long as you desire. Recommended options can be combined in such a way that you always eat an enjoyable, and balanced diet.

Weight and measurements are usually reduced very slowly, but some will lose excess fat very quickly.

The purpose of the Bolio System is not to generate spectacular weight losses, but to teach you to eat in a balanced way and to reduce excess body fat through a healthy plan. Slowly losing weight and inches with a program that includes an abundance of all food groups is a fantastic result, even when only modest losses of weight and measurements are obtained.

Some may regain weight and inches when using this program. In 90% of these cases, this is due to an inadvertent reduction of the consumption of vegetable fats. If you do gain inches, you must first add avocados, almonds, and/or olive oil to your menu. If you add vegetable fats and still continue to gain weight, go back to a week that left you satisfied and clearly resulted in a loss of weight and inches. This way, you can start to lose fat again without having to repeat the program from the first week.

It is also worthwhile to check just how well you are sticking to your plan. During one week write down on a piece of paper just exactly what you are eating as well as the hours you are doing it. You will probably be surprised to find that you are not including all food groups and/or you are not keeping a tight schedule.

Not being disciplined with the program is not a great problem, as long as you take conscience and make the necessary adjustments.

When I published the first edition of this book, my telephone was flooded with calls from people who had reduced excess body fat, but, when moving to the maintenance part of the program, regained part of what they had lost.

This forced me to seek an alternative plan that would favor a permanent reduction of excess body fat.

This option can be found in my book, *What the Naturally Skinny Do to Stay Skinny* (under translation), which has a more structured maintenance technique. If for some reason you have regained part of what you lost, consult that other book since it offers a series of alternatives to Week Eight recommended in this book.

If the present method generated satisfactory loss of body fat, but you feel it is not practical in the long run, I again recommend *What the Naturally Skinny Do to Stay Skinny*. It contains programs for those who usually eat in restaurants. This other book does not offer a new program, but is more an expansion of possibilities.

I have also published a recipe book with menus developed by Mexican Chef Gloria Funtanet. This again is not a substitute for the program outlined in this book, but rather offers further options.

Week Nine?

Are you ready to include in your diet all those tasty dishes that have been avoided in weeks one through eight? Do you feel bold enough to fight face to face with your second greatest enemy? (Your greatest enemies are severely restricted diets).

There is no hurry to face the challenge of saturated fats, since this temptation will always be present in our lives. This is why I put a question mark after "week nine." If you wish to continue with the recommendations for the previous weeks, go ahead.

But it would be naïve to think that you will never again eat food rich in saturated fats. After all, they are a very pleasant part of life. In social settings, in restaurants, at a friend's house, and in many other places, we will be exposed to these food groups. A more sensible and honest attitude is to learn to control and limit the consumption of saturated fats.

When you are ready to face enemy number two, apply one, or all, of the strategies presented in this chapter. There is no precise way to control and limit saturated fats. Of the many techniques that make us eat less, you can use those that are most practical or accessible. Following are several options for controlling and limiting your intake of saturated fats.

TIME

The human body has its own warehouses where it stores whatever is needed for survival. If for some reason we can't eat carbohydrates, we have a reservoir that will protect us for approximately 72 hours. After this time, the body will start using its protein reservoirs (muscle) to compensate for the lack of carbohydrates. The protein warehouse will sustain us for four to six weeks, even if we don't eat any protein. The fat warehouse allows the body to subsist for months without fat in the diet.

It is not necessary that we have all food groups every time we sit down to eat. Ideally we should eat carbohydrates as many times as possible during the day, but fats and protein can be taken only once a day or even once every two or three days without causing any metabolic changes.

Thanks to these reserves, we can eat as much as we want of saturated fats without becoming overweight. This means that you can eat all the pizza or Gouda cheese that you desire and continue losing weight and inches off your measurements. That is, of course, you can do this as long as you eat large amounts of saturated fats preferably on the weekend.

To do this, first reduce the amount of saturated fats you eat on weekdays. This is equal to a vegetarian diet. If you don't fancy a vegetarian diet, select fish, shellfish, non-fat milk, non-fat yogurt, turkey breasts, chicken breasts, or lean steak (Weeks Three to Five) since all these foods contain minimum quantities of saturated fats.

In order for this technique to work, make sure that you eat enough vegetable oils all week long. Remember that olive oil is ideal for cooking and other vegetable oils (such as corn oil) should be eaten uncooked.

This is an excellent technique that allows you to eat all you want on the occasional weekend, as long as you correctly compensate for it on weekdays. This is the option that is most frequently used by my patients.

COMPETITION

Many have the erroneous belief that they must always control what they eat or they will run the risk of bursting from eating too much. They erroneously think that their body has absolutely no way of imposing its own limits when it comes to food.

By now, you should already know that this is false and that your stomach definitely has a limit. This is because our brain measures with precision what we eat, and when we have taken enough, it will notify us that we must stop eating by making us feel full and by making further food seem distasteful or unappealing. This control is present even in the most gluttonous people in the world. The moment will always come when food consumption is spontaneously curtailed, when we "just can't eat any more."

We are armed with a powerful primitive tool of self-control that can help us moderate what we eat, and it's very easy for us to make use of this tool. All you have to do is change the order in which you eat your food.

Do you want to eat less pizza without feeling limited or punished? First drink a large glass of fruit juice or non-diet soft drink, followed by a large salad and a plate of pasta. Then go ahead and eat all you want of that delicious pizza that you ordered. Inverting the order of food groups works quite well. When you leave your most "addictive" dish for last, you can limit its consumption without feeling punished.

This option is fantastic for any type of dessert such as apple pies, doughnuts, etc.

In order for this, or any other, technique to work, you must frequently measure your body. For a three-week test period, measure yourself every other day. This way you can detect when you have eaten excessive quantities of saturated fats. Don't expect immediate effects from a high-fat diet. A well-nourished body defends itself very efficiently from a high-fat diet. Only after two or three weeks of eating excess amounts of fat will you begin to notice an increase in your measurements. If your gain inches, carefully analyze what you have done during the last three weeks. Don't fool yourself into thinking that your bulging waistline is due to yesterday's overindulgence at dinner.

DISPLACEMENT

Since the stomach has a limit, we can fill it with complex carbohydrates and protein, with food high in saturated fats, or with some combination of these.

If you have decided to include foods high in fats, either saturated or heated, tilt the combination toward food high in complex carbohydrates. For example, if you decide to eat a hamburger, eat lots of lettuce and tomato, some avocado and a very large glass of your favorite fruit juice. If possible, eat a plate of beans along with your hamburger.

What do you get from all this? This will make you eat less meat. In the previous technique, dishes high in fats are left until the end of your meal, but this is not always practical. The displacement technique is more flexible. If you include various food groups in the same bite, you will not add excess fat to your body as long as each bite contains more complex carbohydrates than fats.

This option must be carefully monitored through both the scale and the measuring tape. Remember that weighing yourself is not enough since the scale is of limited use in determining the loss or gain of body fat.

Although there are wide variations to the following guidelines, I have found that depending on the nutritional mistake that you fall into you will dictate the region of the body that accumulates fat:

If your hip measurement increases, it is almost certain that you ate too many fats even if you used one of these techniques to limit them.

On the other hand, if your waist measurement increases, be very careful, since this might mean that you are: **not including enough** quantities of fruits, vegetables, legumes, cereals, fats and/or protein in your program; you are **not observing the proper time schedules** for eating; or you are **experiencing chronic and intense stress** in your life; or there is a **combination of all three.**

If thoracic fat is accumulated, this is usually due to the fact that you are not eating every two to three hours, or that you are not observing your time schedules.

FIBER CONSUMPTION

This technique is very, very popular and is quite a simple technique to use, but for some reason few people use it as a permanent strategy.

How does this recommendation work?

It is a variation of the competition technique, but with the small difference that foods with high fiber content and low calorie content are used. Fiber makes you feel full, stays in the stomach longer, and also interferes with fat absorption. Fiber consumption helps you eat high-fat foods without doing too much damage to the body.

Unfortunately, there is one problem with this option; the high fiber meal must be taken 10 to 30 minutes before you sit down to eat the high-fat dish.

Which fiber is best? All are useful. Don't be deceived by publicity into buying products that promise you spectacular results. Use normal foods that are easy to prepare. Here are some examples, but there are many others:

Vegetable smoothie:
cucumber   ½ (small)
pineapple   1 thick slice
fruit juice   6 oz

Blend all ingredients and drink 10 to 30 minutes before a high-fat food.

Psyllium plantago (Metamucil®)	1 tsp. dissolved in water before the high-fat food
Dehydrated cactus (nopal):	1 cup before eating the high-fat food
Any salad:	as much as you want before eating the high-fat food
Boiled beans:	A large plate full before eating the high-fat food.

These techniques are useful as long as you also consume large enough quantities of other nutrients (including vegetable fats). That is to say, they will work as long as you use them only occasionally and you eat a balanced menu the rest of the week.

Remember that excess body fat can also be caused by a very low fat diet, a non balanced diet, and a very low calorie diet. When you eat less than your body needs, sooner or later it triggers the starvation mode. Either malnutrition due to an unbalanced diet or under nutrition due to a severely restricted diet can increase the ability of your body to turn any food group into fat.

Prolonged, sustained fasting will also lead to an increase in body fat, even if you are eating a balanced menu once or twice a day.

In the long run, those who frequently follow very restricted diets only gain more weight, a bigger waistline, and thinner ankles.

Any or all of the techniques described above can be used, and you should apply the technique which is easiest or best suited to your lifestyle. Some may decide to eat saturated fats only once a week. Others may use all of the techniques at the same time. It is only through trial and error that you will be able to define which option or options are best for you.

A final word of caution: a menu high in saturated fats may lead to high cholesterol levels. It is wise to check this possibility with your doctor when you start week nine. Remember that I advise you to review this or any other program with your doctor before, during, and after following the program.

HOW MANY MEALS PER DAY?

One of the hardest habits to maintain is eating many times a day.

It is quite true that fractioning meals helps you lose fat more quickly, but this is not necessarily the eating style that may fit your life patterns.

If eating frequently is almost impossible, try to eat at least four meals per day with a maximum time interval of six hours.

The Last Week

After all these weeks, what follows?

By now, you should have firmly established the following eating pattern: You wake up hungry; you can easily eat a hearty breakfast; during the day, you feel hungry every two to three hours; once you start eating, you quickly feel satisfied; your desire for fruits and vegetables is clear and strong; and food with a high fat content usually generates discomfort or even nausea. Above all, you feel no fear of eating large quantities of any type of food, including carbohydrates and fats.

You should also be able to control your consumption of saturated fats with ease, instead of completely eliminating them. If your fear of food has become fear of fat, at all costs resist the temptation to avoid eating fats altogether.

If, on the contrary, the recommendations have seemed difficult to apply and you are still burdened with old habits, don't worry. This is perfectly normal. Changing any habit is difficult, but not impossible. The human tendency is to unconsciously repeat the same actions again and again and to resist any type of change. This unconscious repetitive behavior is called a habit.

Resistance to change is not caused by some evil motivation buried in our tormented past or unhappy childhood. It is just as difficult to start a new activity, such as an exercise or sensible diet program, as it is to stop doing it once it has become a routine.

Permanent loss of body fat is very difficult to obtain for two reasons. In the first place, we naturally prefer the taste of fatty foods. Secondly, we cannot completely eliminate fats from our diets. Smoking and alcoholism are very straightforward addictions. If you are addicted to tobacco or alcohol, it is safest to avoid them completely. You cannot do this with food fats. If you were foolish enough to attempt this, it would cause very significant health problems and you would almost certainly regain all of the body fat you had lost. That is why you must learn to consume fats in a balanced manner.

Losing excess body fat is indeed a very complicated problem. You must not torture yourself with negative thoughts or conclude that you are a failure or a worthless human being for failing to accomplish this difficult task. If in your first attempt you were unable to strictly follow the Bolio System, you have the obligation to try again. But before repeating the program, carefully analyze the reasons for your poor adherence.

The most important element that influences your ability to change any habit is your lifestyle. Your ability to lose body fat, like other aspects of your life, is influenced by your workload, your significant other, family interaction, personal expectations, your emotions, and many other factors that are unique for each person.

From time to time, it is wise to ask for the professional help of a psychologist, who will support you in making permanent changes in your life. This does not mean you will have to spend years in psychoanalysis before you have any hope of becoming thin. It certainly does not imply spending hours mourning over past events. The purpose of psychological counseling is to help you increase your self-esteem, define your goals more precisely, and improve your motivation.

It doesn't matter why you grew fat, whether the reason is metabolic or emotional or both. The important thing to keep in mind is that you have to start working efficiently to solve the problem.

Since fear of food is sometimes difficult to eradicate, I developed the *Changing Dietary Habits Workshop*. It has been presented in different health institutions, including the Institute of Social Security (in Mexico), the office of the Secretary of Health (Mexico's governmental health institution), the Pan-American Health Organization (a branch of the World Health Organization), and UNICEF. This workshop is currently being offered in Mexico's major medical centers.

On the other hand, those of you who have found following the Bolio System a "picnic" or "a piece of cake" should not fall into the error of believing that you have forever eradicated your problem. You still face the challenge of remaining slender till the last week of your life.

If you obtained satisfactory results, use this last week to apply all you have learned and establish a personal nutritional plan. You now know the theory and have correctly practiced eating a balanced diet at all times. Now you have the responsibility of transforming these habits into a permanent eating style.

According to international reports, almost 90% relapse within the first three months of finishing fat-loss treatments. Therefore, you should be constantly alert to the way you eat for at least one year.

Why should excess body fat return?

International studies indicate that the most frequent association with relapse is emotional conflict. If you have successfully changed how you eat, take extra care in stressful times. When you lower your guard during conflict and other difficult situations, you run the risk of falling back into an inappropriate eating pattern.

Surely some of you who have followed the Bolio System will have obtained spectacular changes in your figure. Others perhaps will have noticed only modest but still satisfactory reductions. It is also possible that some of you have seen no changes at all. Those who still have significant amounts of excess body fat in spite of applying all recommendations with self-discipline and enthusiasm should read with great care the following pages.

PART FOUR
ANY QUESTIONS?

The Plateau
(Why do I sometimes stop losing weight and inches?)

How marvelous it would be to lose excess body fat at the same rate from the first to the last day of any program!

Unfortunately, not even absolute fasting generates such uniform changes. At first, you lose weight and inches very quickly. Later, your weight loss slows down, and finally a time comes when you lose nothing at all or may even gain back some of what you have lost.

The human body needs a certain amount of time to get used to a new environment. It has been calculated that when you lose fat, at least 80 enzymatic reactions are modified. When your body adapts to this new environment, you stop losing weight, and this is called a "plateau."

In recent years, many studies of this phenomenon have been carried out. Here are some of the primary conclusions:

1. Changes are never the same. Some people lose weight quickly, while others lose nothing at all. The rate of fat loss even changes in the same person with the same diet. That is to say, the diet that didn't work for you today may produce spectacular changes tomorrow, and vice versa. These variations occur regardless of the type of diet, the individual's faithfulness in adhering to the diet, or the length of time the person has been on the diet.

2. When you do lose weight and inches, the changes come intermittently, in a pattern characterized by alternating periods of reduction and plateau.

3. A plateau will generally last from two to four weeks. Once 20 pounds of body fat have been lost, the plateaus become more prolonged and can last from two to six months.

4. The maximum amount of fat that can safely be lost at one time is 20 pounds which amounts to three inches off your body's measurements.

Once this goal is achieved, it is best to wait some time (two to six months) before trying to lose more fat.

5. Reductions of more than 20 pounds at a rapid and uniform rate will usually produce severe metabolic changes that favor the regaining of lost fat. (That is, your body, sensing the rapid weight loss, will make adjustments so that it uses food much more efficiently, to the point that you may start to gain weight.)

6. Above all, you must remain patient and avoid the yo-yo syndrome of constantly gaining and losing weight. Repeated weight fluctuations due to diets will in the long run do more damage than just being overweight, since the resulting increases in abdominal fat can lead to diabetes, hypertension, elevated cholesterol and triglyceride levels (and, consequently, a heart attack), and pre-senile dementia.

7. If you need to lose more than 20 pounds, you should be mentally and emotionally prepared to make important and permanent changes to your lifestyle, in which a balanced diet is accompanied by at least 30 minutes of physical activity every day.

8. Lesser weight reductions are usually explained by failure to adhere to the program. If you have strictly and carefully carried out all recommendations of the Bolio System, the absence of fat loss may be due to a stressful lifestyle. Diets and stress do not go together well.

9. Those who have spent many years dieting will notice that with every new diet, fat loss becomes more and more difficult to achieve. This is explained by the increased metabolic efficiency unleashed by those same diets. More than a diet, these people need a sensible, balanced program which includes an abundance of good food and which will help them develop a healthy, well-nourished body. In my experience, once this is obtained, fat loss will occur spontaneously.

10. Recent research has reported that cold weather may favor fat accumulation. In my personal experience, people using the Bolio System will lose less fat during winter, and more fat during spring, than during any other season of the year. You must take this into account when starting the program in

cold months. Christmas is an especially interesting time, since festivities around this date are closely associated with special dishes.

Above all, you must be patient and disciplined in order to achieve the objective of permanently eliminating excess body fat. Common sense will tell you that there are no magic potions or miraculous cures in the battle to eradicate excess body fat.

Questions and Answers

Until now, I have been writing as if you had all the time in the world to apply the Bolio System, never had difficulty following any recommendation, never went on vacation, did not know temptation, did not have to feed a family, had perfectly educated children and never ate in restaurants.

If you are not so lucky and do possess some human traits, you will surely have many questions concerning how to correctly follow all recommendations.

In the following pages, I will answer questions that are frequently asked concerning the Bolio System. If I fail to answer a specific question, send it by mail or e-mail to the addresses noted at the end of this chapter.

How much weight and how many inches can I lose if I correctly apply all of the recommendations?

In traditional strategies that try to eliminate body fat by reducing the amount of food eaten, approximately 20% do not observe any changes, and 8% gain weight. That is to say, there is close to a 30% failure rate with the usual weight-loss programs.

With the Bolio System, I have managed to reduce the failure rate, but 12% of those who undertake the program still see no weight change, and 3% gain weight.

Why is this? It is a response influenced by many factors such as age; gender; how long the person has been overweight; the degree of malnutrition; heredity; the number of diets the person has been on previously; the type of physical activity the person is involved in; the degree of stress the person is experiencing; the time of year; the presence of other health problems such as diabetes, high uric acid, high cholesterol, and high triglycerides; and the person's level of adherence to recommendations.

Who will quickly lose excess fat? An 18-to-40-year-old male who has been overweight for less than five years; has little or no malnutrition; has no overweight relatives; has never been on a diet; is involved in moderate physical activity; is experiencing little stress; starts this program in spring; has normal levels of blood glucose, cholesterol, triglycerides, and uric acid; and has the will power of a saint in following the plan's recommendations.

Who will lose excess fat slowly, or even gain weight and inches? A woman who is more than 40 years old; has been overweight for more than five years; is malnourished; has overweight relatives; has been on one diet or another most of her life; is engaged in either excessive or no physical activity; is constantly stressed; starts this programs in winter; has elevated levels of glucose, cholesterol, triglycerides, and uric acid; and is undisciplined in following the recommendations of the program.

Which list are you in? Most of the characteristics that put you in one list or the other cannot be changed. For example, those who have been on weight-loss diets most of their lives cannot erase their past. Neither is it possible to change the fact that you have been overweight for more than five years or that you have overweight relatives.

You should face squarely the reality of these characteristics that affect the speed of weight loss, but you should not let them discourage you. It is time to stop living in a fairy tale world, thinking you can find a magic solution to the problem of excess body fat.

On the Bolio System, 20% lose more than 1 ½ pounds per week, 50% lose one pound per week, 15% lose less than one pound per week, 12% see no change, and 3% experience increases in their weight and measurements.

If you have gained weight and inches in the first two weeks of the program, up to two pounds and/or half an inch on your measurements, don't despair. You will generally lose them when applying the rest of the plan. Be patient and fight through the frustration of not losing, or even gaining, some weight at first.

If you gain more than two pounds, stop the program and seek help from a weight-control specialist, who will help you eat without gaining weight.

You must have the perseverance of an experienced hunter stalking a difficult prey if you wish to succeed in losing excess body fat.

What should I do if I am currently on another diet or weight-loss program?

The only guarantee that you have when applying a strict diet that makes you lose weight quickly is that you will regain all your lost weight as soon as you go off the diet. If you are also taking some medication to burn fat, you may even experience rebound (a spectacular gain of more weight than was lost).

In order to reduce or prevent the rebound effect, apply the *Recovery Phase* (see weeks one and two). I have sometimes seen impressive losses of weight and inches in people who started the Recovery Phase after being on a low-carbohydrate diet.

What should I do if, instead of losing weight, I gain it?

The first thing is to not despair. This does not mean that the Bolio System is useless, or that you have been cursed to always be overweight. Weight gain in these circumstances is almost always secondary to malnutrition. When you are severely malnourished, you greatly increase your risk of gaining weight and inches with *any changes made to your usual eating habits*. The irony of this situation is that only those who have very carefully and methodically followed strict recommendations of previous weight-loss plans will suffer from severe malnutrition.

Why is this so? Because nobody in his right mind, except for the very disciplined, would starve when surrounded by tasty and healthy food. This does not mean that you should frequently repeat the first two weeks of the Bolio System (the Recovery Phase). You will slowly lose excess fat on this plan and do not need to repeat those introductory weeks.

The sensible attitude for those who have been on weight-loss diets most of their lives is to have extraordinary patience and wait for their bodies to reduce excess fat when their bodies decide to do so.

Remember that if you gain more than two pounds of weight despite applying the program with precision, you must suspend it and seek help from an obesity expert.

What should I do if I frequently eat in restaurants?

The greatest obstacle to following this book is food eaten outside of your home. Besides eating in restaurants, problems occur when feasting on special occasions (such as birthdays and holidays) and when eating at the house of a friend who is not following recommendations of the Bolio System. However, some people complain that the greatest difficulty is at home, when the official cook, usually the mother or wife, refuses to prepare the "insipid" dishes recommended in this program.

When you have little or no control over how food is prepared, how can you succeed in reducing excess body fat? Several options exist, but before applying any of these recommendations, check your triglyceride levels and review these options with your physician.

Most restaurants offer low-fat menus, which are usually very tasty and balanced. But remember to ask for a low-fat, not a low-calorie, menu. Eat these low-fat menu items as often as you can for one week and check your measurements.

If your waist and hip measurements are decreasing, this means that the restaurant's low-fat menu is good for you. But if your waist measurements increase, this means that you are taking insufficient fats and must add vegetable fats (olive oil, nuts, avocados, etc.) to your restaurant menu, or at another time in the day.

On the other hand, if your thigh measurements are increasing, this means that your "low-fat" diet has more fats than your body needs. In this case, assume you are getting all your daily fat rations at the restaurant. This will force you to eat no fats the rest of the day (drink non fat milk, eat boiled pasta, fresh fruits, vegetables, whole grain bread, etc.).

I will phrase this in another way: mal nutrition and/or under nutrition will usually accumulate fat in and around the waist, while accumulation of fat in hips and glutei is generally secondary to a high fat diet.

If you see no change in your measurements, or even slowly regain some of what you had lost, use any of the techniques recommended in week nine. The most practical technique is competition, eating carbohydrates and/or a high-fiber food group. In restaurants, have your fruit juice with whole grain bread before starting your main course. On festive occasions (or when eating at a friend's home) ask for a glass of fruit juice before eating anything else. If you feel comfortable doing this, ask the host to prepare some fruit and/or a vegetable plate that you can eat before the main menu.

Another option is to request, as much as possible, food prepared with little or no fat. Talk to the cook at a restaurant where you eat frequently and ask for a non-fat or low-fat dish. Perhaps the first time you do this, your request will seem strange. By the tenth time you request a special plate, perhaps you will be asked what you are doing to lose excess fat.

You also have the option of balancing the regular high-fat menu at a restaurant with what you eat the rest of the day. If you have a special routine, such as eating a hamburger or pizza every day at a certain restaurant (something I do not recommend), contact me through my website for advice on what to eat the rest of the day so that you at least do not gain excess fat. The address is: www.drbolio.com or www.esbelto.com (Spanish version).

At home, the solution might be simple: Ask whoever does the cooking to have a plate of fruit ready for you when you get home. When you arrive, eat fruits and vegetables, and, if you wish, have a glass of fruit juice. Then, when you sit down at the table, you won't be as hungry and will be able to eat whatever dish is served, plus more fruit and vegetables and whole grain bread. If the plate of vegetables and fruit is not ready when you get home, you can always prepare it yourself. Remember that you are the one on diet. If your family forbids you to eat fruit and vegetables before sitting down at the table, look for professional support to help you manage such a destructive relationship.

When you are invited to a friend's house, be polite and offer to bring a special low-fat or non-fat dish. You can take boiled rice, or some other such dish. If you don't have time or don't know how to cook, buy a salad at a vegetarian restaurant or an appropriate plate of Japanese food.

If you need to negotiate at home, you have several weapons to help you obtain what you want: Ask for a low-fat dish in exchange for a well-kept room or perhaps an invitation to the movies.

It is crucial that your loved ones understand how important it is for you to remain slender. If at first they do not pay attention, accept it. It is understandable that they don't believe in what you are doing, especially if you already have had a long history of being on diets. If you are persistent and show them how you eliminate excess fat while eating all kinds of food, all the while maintaining an excellent state of mind and good health, surely the moment will arrive when they will want to share this nutritious program with you. But if you are in a bad mood when following the Bolio System's recommendations, don't blame them if they ask, or even demand, that you stop such foolishness and start enjoying life again without tormenting yourself about food.

What should I do if I am so hungry that I can't follow recommendations?

You should never feel hungry. If you're hungry, it means that recommendations for the week that you are in are insufficient and you must move up to a week with more food; that is, instead of starting with the low-calorie menus, begin with the higher-calorie menus (week five and on).

The worse that could happen when doing this is triggering the re-feeding phenomenon with subsequent weight gain. Although this has no relationship with body fat accumulation, it will usually provoke panic, especially if you are obsessed with the scale.

Therefore, you must decide which will be more intolerable: a feeling of hunger that will disappear as the program goes on or the possibility of gaining weight but not inches. To make your decision easier, always keep in mind that the intention of this program is not to focus on the scale in the short run, but to teach you to eat in such a healthy way that you will never gain weight again.

What should I do if for some reason I did not follow recommendations very well?

A satisfactory response is obtained when you follow 70% or more of recommendations. Greater adherence will result in better results. But it is possible that over twelve weeks you will encounter situations that will limit your ability to correctly apply all recommendations. Perhaps you will become ill and have no time to prepare your food, or perhaps it will be difficult to obtain certain elements of the program.

Excess body fat is accumulated when you eat a high-fat diet. But it can also be appear with prolonged fasting and/or malnutrition. Excess body fat caused by malnutrition is more harmful and more difficult to eradicate than excess body fat caused by a high-fat diet. If you cannot apply a balanced program, eat what is at hand. It is preferable that you eat what you can find than to expose yourself to malnutrition. Always try to include fruits, vegetables, cereals, and legumes, but if this option does not exist, have sweets, chocolates, French fries, or even junk food. If at all possible, prefer vegetable fats such as avocado and nuts over other types of fat. And then, of course, do this only for small periods of time. It is very important that you do not stop eating, and, above all, don't feel frustrated because you can only select high-fat food at a particular meal.

What should your attitude be? Enjoy what you are eating, and plan better for the next occasion.

Not losing weight or inches because you haven't been able to follow the program perfectly isn't terrible, as long as you recognize where you fall short and learn to eat without fear in unexpected circumstances.

Now, if these "emergencies" appear every other day of the week, it would be wise to obtain help from a professional or from self help group such as Overeaters Anonymous.

What should I do if I have a craving?

Don't worry. When cravings hit, eat the food that you crave, but in such a way that it does not cause digestive symptoms. That is, savor a little of the food, but don't gorge yourself on it. My philosophy is that cravings should please your palate and that nutritious food should fill your stomach. Once you have eaten a small portion of the food you crave, whether it is chocolate or French fries continue with all recommendations in the Bolio System. Do not substitute what you craved for some food group on the menu, for as long as you follow the program, occasional cravings will never cause fat accumulation.

A word of caution, if you give in to your cravings and find out that you ate so much that you cannot continue with recommended meals, it usually means that you are punishing your usual daily caloric intake. Therefore you must **immediately** advance to a higher week that gives you more food. This will help you to easily control any new craving.

I will say it another way: overindulgence of cravings must be solved by eating **more healthy foods and not less**.

How much water should I drink?

We need two to three liters of water per day, and in hot climates even more. The menus in the Bolio System already include between one and two liters of water. Therefore you can add extra water by taking four to eight cups of water per day. High quantities of water are useless in a weight-loss program, but they do help improve digestion. The menus in this program are very high in fiber, and water will help fiber work correctly.

You can add tea (green tea probably helps you lose excess fat), coffee, water with lemon, or just plain water.

I do not recommend artificially flavored water *or any other type of "diet" drinks or meals*. Remember that you are allowed to add any extra snack that you desire as long as you eat all marked meals. This includes normally sweetened drinks.

Also remember that you must re-learn to eat all foods groups (including the ones associates to excess body fat) to consider yourself cured of this problem.

Can I consume coffee or tea?

In relation to excess body fat, there is no reason you should not enjoy these drinks, but you should keep in mind that certain ailments, such as fibrocystic mastopathy (lumps in the breast), may be made worse by these beverages. If you have any doubts, have your doctor check you and decide what is best.

Recent reports suggest that taking more than five cups of coffee per day may favor fat accumulation. On the other hand, drinking green tea may help you shed excess pound and protect you from ischemic cardiopathy (a reduction of blood flow to the heart).

Can I consume alcoholic beverages?

Avoiding alcohol during the first three weeks of this program is essential, since, as intoxication rises, motivation is reduced. After the third week, you can drink whisky, tequila, vodka, or cognac. These beverages have low quantities of free radicals. Although wine has more free radicals than previous alcoholic beverages, it may help you reduce cholesterol and risk of heart attack in moderate amounts.

If you find it impossible to avoid alcoholic beverages for three weeks, seriously consider the possibility that your social alcoholism has become an addiction.

How long should I feel guilty for not following the program's recommendations?

No more than five minutes.

Feelings of guilt help us detect attitudes or situations that should be changed in our lives. Without this feeling, we would probably have little capacity to correct mistakes. But tormenting yourself with guilt for days on end is useless.

An exaggerated feeling of guilt can cause two totally different problems. In the first place, we can spend so much time feeling guilty that we will not have enough time or energy to change our habits; regretting errors is one way of avoiding change. Second, we can feel so guilty that we decide to make our own personal alterations to the program and refuse to eat some of the recommended foods. This only causes malnutrition and the risk of accumulating more body fat.

If you are a perfectionist, take great care. Food is useful, among others things, for obtaining pleasure in life. If you are extremely anxious to follow every last detail of the recommendations, you will limit your ability to enjoy food. This will condemn your fat-loss efforts to failure, since it is almost impossible to make an unpleasant task a habit.

If necessary, repeat to yourself a thousand times that excess body fat is solved with patience and wisdom and that, just like any other human being, you will make mistakes in following recommendations of this program.

What strategy should I follow on holidays?

The best recommendation is to forget that diets exist.

On holidays, our daily tensions are usually reduced. This favors the loss of excess body fat, even when you don't follow any recommendation (unless of course, you're so severely malnourished that *any* extra meal will make you gain weight and inches). This is the best way to demonstrate the impact of chronic stress upon excess body fat.

On holidays also, physical activity is usually increased; we walk, swim, dance, etc., which favors a reduction in body fat as long as exercise is moderate.

Here is the most important reason for not following your program at these times: On vacations, you generally have little control over how food is prepared. If you try to avoid high-fat food, it will almost always result in an unbalanced diet. This may only lead to gaining fat due to malnutrition.

If (in the worst case scenario) you are going to gain excess weight while on vacation, it is better that you obtain it from eating more and not from eating less; excess body fat secondary to a high-fat diet responds more quickly than excess fat due to malnutrition.

My main caution is that you eat whatever is at hand as many times as you can each day (remember that eating frequently protects you from the accumulation of body fat) and that you enjoy it. This is the ideal moment to listen to your body and give it what it asks for.

It is wise to include dried fruits in your suitcase and eat them when waking up, before going to sleep, and, especially on prolonged trips, during the day. Remember that adding nuts to fruit will reduce the glycemic index.

Eat whatever you desire (soft drinks, ice cream, snacks, fresh fruit, etc.) as frequently as possible. This will help you reach breakfast, lunch, and dinner without feeling hungry or famished. Our worst enemy on vacations is excessive hunger.

Do whatever is necessary to have at least three main meals a day.

Most importantly: Intensely enjoy your holidays.

Can I follow the plan if I have diabetes?

The Bolio System causes favorable changes in diabetics, generally leading to excellent control of blood glucose. In many cases diabetics may reduce or even suspend their medication. But it is indispensable that you obtain the approval of your doctor and that you apply recommendations under strict medical supervision, since blood glucose will usually be reduced and there is a slight risk of hypoglycemia (a reduction of blood glucose), and this can cause severe damage to your organs.

Unfortunately, you will not see great changes in your weight or inches until your glucose level falls below 160 milligrams per deciliter. This also holds true for high levels of cholesterol and/or triglycerides. You will only lose inches when these levels are normalized. Following the Bolio System will reduce or help control all three factors. Therefore, your first objective when following the plan is to reduce these elements instead of eliminating excess body fat. Loss of body fat will ensue when underlying problems are controlled.

High levels of previously marked elements do not always produce symptoms and the best way to establish levels is through laboratory tests. If you are more than 30 years old, you should get glucose, triglyceride, and cholesterol levels checked every year, whether or not on diet. Younger people should have tests only if there is family history of these problems or are unable to lose weight or inches when following the Bolio System.

If you have these or any other medical problem, it does not mean you should suspend the Bolio System, but neither is the plan a substitute for medical care. Use your common sense and review with your doctor the possibility of using this or any other program.

Can I follow recommendations during pregnancy?

All of my books are designed for the general population. During pregnancy, there are special requirements depending on which month of gestation the woman is in. Even though the Bolio System constitutes an excellent nutritional program, the best option for pregnant women is to follow an individualized program. Only with your doctor's approval should you follow this or any other program.

Weight loss is so evident and results are usually so spectacular that gynecologists will almost always worry about the baby's development. I can assure you that this program favors the growth of perfectly normal children, but then again, it is your doctor's decision as to what kind of nutritional recommendations you should follow *and* what laboratory tests he may need to follow your pregnancy.

Can I follow the program if I am breast-feeding?

Here is great news for post-partum women: spectacular changes in weight and measurements can be obtained as long as you eat an abundant and balanced plan. The response to this program is so spectacular for post-partum women that I call it the "metabolic window." If you are also breast-feeding, the response is even better. According to the World Health Organization you must eat no less than 1500 calories per day (that is, follow the recommendations for week five or higher), and I personally recommend starting with 2000 calories or more (week seven). You must also take into account that breast-feeding imposes extra requirements for elements such as iron and calcium. Therefore, I strongly insist that you review week six or seven of this program with your doctor or dietitian.

What if I had a caesarean?

Caesarean section, as well as any other surgical procedure, causes a special response known as "surgical stress." Nutritional needs are highly increased, but unfortunately appetite is curtailed. Therefore, even in the best of cases, you should expect to add an inch to your measurements within four weeks after any surgery (it makes no difference whether it is an appendectomy or caesarean). You can minimize this phenomenon by eating a balanced diet of at least 2000 calories per day after your surgeon permits it. This is the calorie level for week seven, but you must first obtain approval of your doctor, or, better yet, ask your dietitian to design a special balanced program that adapts to recommendations of this book.

Can children follow recommendations of the program?

The Bolio System is an excellent tool to ingrain healthy eating habits in children while providing nutritious and tasty food. However, it is important to remember that children from age two on need more than 1500 calories per day or they will run the risk of stunting their growth. This calorie level is obtained from the menus recommended for week five and following. But it is indispensable that you first obtain the consent of yourh doctor and that he closely monitors any changes.

When you obtain your doctor's consent to follow these recommendations, remember that the suggested meals are only a guideline and that your child can, and should, eat all food groups. That is to say, children can and must add any food they want, as long as they comply with 70% or more of the recommendations.

Just as with pregnancy, where obese mothers will almost always lose weight without blunting the growth of their offspring, pediatrics specialists will be surprised with the results of this program, since children will usually lose weight, inches around the waist *and* gain inches in height at the same time.

Can I follow the program if I am already skinny?

I have known sad stories of thin people who started diets because of vanity, and ended up becoming overweight because of metabolic alterations triggered by those diets. Skinny people can start with recommendations of weeks five through seven. In a permanent and healthy way, they will lose whatever small accumulations of excess fat they have while gaining firmer buttocks. Women will usually obtain more beautiful breasts, especially with week seven. This can be achieved without risking malnutrition. Thin people do not need to apply weeks one through four of the program. The aesthetic changes caused by the Bolio System are excellent in people with excess fat, and extraordinary in thin individuals.

In one of Mexico's major hospitals, I prescribed a balanced 3,000-calorie diet to 20 thin and healthy women workers who were not on diet and had maintained a stable weight for more than one year. My intention was to demonstrate that even women with normal weight would lose abdominal fat while eating an overabundant and balanced menu. To my surprise, they increased their breast size and consistency, their gluteus (buttocks) became more rounded, and they lost inches from their waists. I concluded that their usual eating habits had been limiting their ability to have a more aesthetic body.

Do almonds and/or cashews produce acne?

Many specialists state that there is no relationship between what you eat and acne, but it is important that your family doctor review the nutritional recommendations of this program and make any changes that he or she considers appropriate to solve this problem. In my experience, I have seen some people develop acne when eating cashews and/or almonds. If this is your situation, exchange nuts for olive oil: 1 tsp. or 5 milliliters for every eight almonds or cashews.

Can I apply the program if I am weight lifting?

Weight lifting imposes special nutritional demands that can interfere with the loss of body fat. On the other hand, those who lift weights can use supplements that favor the gain of muscle and at the same time loss of body fat. These supplements generate spectacular results but should be used carefully in accordance with personal needs.

For those lifting weights, I usually recommend a diet composed of 53% carbohydrates, 20% protein, and 27% total fat. In my personal experience, with this combination, muscle will usually become defined and grow faster than with regular recommendations. This may also help ensure a stable change; that is, if for any reason the weight lifting routine is stopped, muscle mass will be maintained for some time. I highly recommend that you seek the professional council of a nutritionist or dietician.

Can I repeat the Recovery Phase (weeks one and two)?

When people read recommendations of week one, they consider them a real challenge. But once they have completed the week, many are so happy with results that they want to apply it again. I know a lady who lost 60 kilograms (about 120 pounds) by constantly repeating recommendations of week two.

The main problem with very strict diets is that they reduce muscle mass along with body fat.

If there was a strategy that quickly burned body fat while sparing muscle mass, it would be acclaimed as an extraordinary strategy to eradicate excess body fat. The *Recovery Phase* (weeks one and two) of the Bolio System qualifies; it quickly reduces excess fat and body fluids and causes little or no loss of muscle.

But even though it offers one of the best methods to burn fat, the *Recovery Phase* does not eliminate excess body fat. Why? Because it has no relationship with normal eating patterns. It is extraordinary for burning fat and providing a quick loss of weight and inches, but it does not teach you to eat. To achieve a stable loss of body fat, it is indispensable that you learn to do it by eating all kinds of food in a prudent and balanced way.

The *Recovery Phase* offered in weeks one and two is of great help in reducing excess fat, but its inappropriate use can cause more damage than benefit. Following are a list of precautions that must be observed if you want to avoid using the technique inappropriately and suffering the rebound effect, regaining more weight than you have lost.

1. Repeat the *Recovery Phase* no more often than once every three months, preferably once every four months. If you repeat it more often, you will surely observe minimal or no changes to your body fat. The human body necessarily eliminates excess fat slowly. Let your body, and not your mind, dictate the speed of weight loss.

Before using the *Recovery Phase again,* follow the maintenance menu for at least four weeks. This way, you will start the *Recovery Phase* with a well-nourished body. The better nourished you are, the quicker the results will be. But if you use this plan a second time and see no results, be very careful. This can mean that the maintenance plan you pursued was more of a malnutrition strategy.

2. Avoid as much as possible using the *Recovery Phase* around Christmas. Trying to lose weight in this season is not a good idea. It is not worth the effort since it will result only in small changes in your figure–in winter, any technique results in less fat loss than it would in the spring. Be patient and wait for spring.

3. Before starting, make sure you have enough time to complete weeks one and two without interruption. If you stop the program part way through, you run the risk of regaining what you have lost.

4. Be disciplined in following recommendations. The most frequent error when repeating the *Recovery Phase* is that you don't follow recommendations as closely as you did the first time. Because you have already lost considerable fat, it is easy to be less strict. This in itself is not serious, as long as you are aware of what you are doing and do not blame the program if you experience minimal or no changes. Usually those who did not lose weight or inches on the first occasion, may see changes the second time.

5. Do not try to force a reduction of more than 20 pounds of fat, or three inches. To stubbornly try to lose more will only trigger the rebound effect. Once you have lost three inches, wait at least two months before trying to lose more weight.

When the *Recovery Phase* is going to be effective, the first results should be seen in 72 hours. If you follow the program correctly and don't obtain promising results in that time, suspend it. Wait at least another month before attempting a new weight loss. This way, you will achieve a gentle loss of fat. There will not be spectacular losses, but neither will you experience painful and frustrating weight regains.

What can I do if I have to lose more than 20 pounds of fat?

After you have lost 20 pounds of fat, and/or three inches off your measurements, your body will almost always experience a plateau, making even the strictest diet ineffective.

Once you have reached a plateau, it is wise to continue with the maintenance program, which includes a balanced menu of all food groups. Stay on the maintenance program for two to three months before attempting another reduction. Then you can repeat the *Recovery Phase* and continue with the rest of the plan exactly as it is presented.

But there are other options: Start with week three, and fill in your extra needs with as many protein shakes as you desire. You can also start with the week that left you feeling satisfied but not overly so. For women, week five is usually sufficient, while men may need week six or seven.

A stricter program will result in faster losses. But keep in mind that violent losses almost always leave an unstable metabolism.

Also remember that once you have lost another three inches, you must suspend your rigid menu and continue with a more open program for at least two months.

I have seen how, using this stair-step approach, patients have lost up to 120 pounds of body fat without gaining them back.

What is the most important element in a successful weight-control program? Patience.

What can I do if I still have doubts?

I am sure that some readers will still have many doubts concerning how to correctly apply recommendations of this program, or perhaps some aspects of this book have seemed confusing. I have tried to write as clearly as possible, but many will probably be reading this type of information for the first time in their life.

It is said that when you read a book, only 10% of the information stays with you. Also, any new knowledge requires time to be understood and adequately handled. Read this book at least three times before starting the program, and once more when you have finished the program.

If your motivation falters, read this book a fifth or sixth time. Many readers tell me they have benefited from reading this document on multiple occasions.

If you read this book at least three times and still find ideas that are not clear, I invite you to write to me. Let me know your doubts, your opinions, your comments, and especially your personal response to this program.

The website address is: www.drbolio.com or www.esbelto.com (Spanish version).

The postal address is:

Dr. Rafael Bolio
PO Box 720298
Miami, FL 33172

APPENDIX
SERVINGS LIST

This list will help you add variety to your daily menu. Once you are comfortable with the program, you can use the list presented below to change any serving indicated in the program. You will find a "new" category in legumes. This is certainly not standard criteria, but it will help you develop a more exact and personalized menu.

CEREAL AND BREAD SERVINGS

A cereal or bread serving contains about 2g of proteins, 16g of carbohydrates, less than 1g of fat and 80 Kilocalories.

CEREALS	AMOUNT
Bran flakes (40%)	½ cup
Ready to eat cereals	¾ cup
Cooked Cereal	½ cup
Cooked Rice	½ cup
Cooked Barley	½ cup
Cooked Pasta	½ cup
Cooked Macaroni	½ cup
Cooked Noodles	½ cup
Cooked Vermicelli	½ cup
Cooked Spaghetti	½ cup
Oatmeal, cooked	½ cup
Pop corn (toasted without oil)	3 cups
Corn Flour	2 tablespoons
Wheat Germ	4 tablespoons

BREAD	AMOUNT
Bread	1 slice (1 oz)
Bread, barley	1 slice (1 oz)
Bread, black	1 oz
Bread, Cuban	1 oz
Bread, pita	1 oz
Bread, rye	1 oz
Bread, soy	1 oz
Bread w/ raisins	1 slice (1 oz)
Bread, whole wheat	1 slice (1 oz)
Bread sticks	½ oz
Crackers, animal	½ oz
Crackers, graham	½ oz
Crackers, matzo	½ oz
Crackers, milk	½ oz
Crackers, Nabisco, wheat thins	½ oz
Crackers, Nabisco, Ritz, low fat	½ oz
Crackers, saltine	6 each
Hamburger roll	1 oz
Hot dog roll	1 oz
Pancake	1 (4" diameter) or 38g
Toast	1 slice (23g)
Tortilla	1 each (1 oz)
Waffle	1 oz

FRUIT SERVINGS:

A fruit serving contains about 12g of carbohydrates, less than 1g of protein and 50 Kilocalories.

FRUIT	AMMOUNT
Apple, medium	½ each
Banana, medium	½ each
Cherries	10 each
Dates	2 each
Figs, dried, uncooked	1 each
Grapefruit, medium	½ each
Grapes	15 each
Kiwi	1 each
Mango	½ cup
Melon	1 cup
Orange	½ cup
Papaya	1 cup
Passion fruit	¼ cup
Pear, medium	½ each
Prune	2 each
Raspberry	¾ cup
Raisins	25 each
Strawberry, sliced	1 cup
Tangerine	½ cup
Watermelon	1 cup

NON FAT MILK SERVINGS:

A Non fat Milk serving contains about 8g of protein, 12g of carbohydrates and 80 Kilocalories.

MILK	PORTION
Non fat milk	8 fl oz
Non fat plan yogurt	5 fl oz

LEGUME SERVING

A legume serving contains about 7g of protein, 20g of carbohydrates and 110 Kilocalories

LEGUME	PORTION
String beans	1 cup
Black beans, mature seeds, cooked	½ cup
Chickpeas, nature seeds, cooked	½ cup
Lentils, mature seed, cooked	½ cup
Broad beans (fava beans)	¾ cup
Small red beans, mature seeds, cooked	½ cup
Soy bean (mature seed) cooked	¾ cup

LEAN PROTEIN SERVINGS

A lean protein serving contains about 8g of protein, 1g or less than fat and 45 Kilocalories.

PROTEIN	PORTION
American cheese, non fat	1 oz
Beef, top round, lean cut, cooked	1 oz
Chicken breast skin not eaten	1 oz
Cottage cheese, low fat	2 oz
Egg white, cooked	3 oz
Fish, cooked	1 ½ oz
Mozzarella cheese, non fat	1 oz
Octopus, cooked	1 oz
Pork, tenderloin, cooked	1 oz
Salmon, cooked	1 oz
Shellfish, cooked (shrimp, lobster, etc.)	1 oz
Swiss cheese, low fat	1 oz
Tuna, light, canned in water	1 oz
Turkey breast, skin not eaten	1 oz
Beef steak, lean	1 oz
Veal cutlet or steak, broiled	1 oz

SUGAR SERVINGS

A sugar serving contains about 4g of carbohydrates and 16 Kilocalories

SUGAR	SERVING
Honey	1 tsp.
Marmalade, all flavors	1 tsp.
Sugar	1 tsp.
Sugar, raw	1 tsp.
Sugar, maple	1 tsp.
Sugar, brown	1 tsp.

FAT SERVINGS

A fat serving (animal or vegetable) contains about 5g of fat and 50 Kilocalories

ANIMAL FAT	SERVING
Butter	1 tsp.
Sour cream	1 oz
Lard	1 tsp.
Bacon strip, meatless	½ oz

VEGETABLE FAT	SERVING
Acorn nuts, dried	½ oz
Avocado, California	1 oz
Avocado, Florida	2 oz
Almonds	8 each
Brazil nuts	¼ oz
Cashew nuts	7 kernels
Hickory nuts	3 each
Mayonnaise, regular	¼ oz (½ tbsp.)
Olives	1 oz
Peanuts, roasted	12 each
Pecans	5 halves
Pine nuts	1/3 oz
Pistachios	14 kernels
Vegetable oil, all types	1 tsp.
Walnuts	4 halves